Food Combining

Better Health — The Natural Way

by Rita Bingham

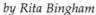

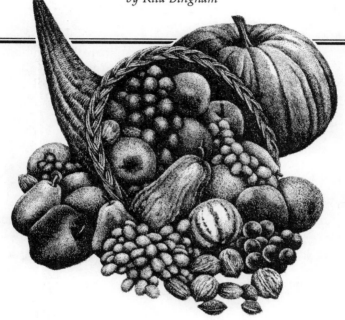

NATURAL MEALS PUBLISHING

Edmond, Oklahoma

ISBN 1-882314-15-8
80 pp. $7.95

Published by Natural Meals Publishing, Edmond, Oklahoma.

Website: www. naturalmeals.com
E-mail: info@naturalmeals.com
OR sales@naturalmeals.com

Fax: 405.359.3492
Order Line: 888.232.6706

Printed in United States of America

Illustrations by Clair Bingham

For my children and grandchildren, to encourage them to seek better health through wholesome foods.

Special Thanks to:

My husband and best friend, Clair, for his great artwork and excellent advice and counsel;

Our daughters Ginni, Kimm, and (daughter-in-law) Rachel, for their help in proofreading and evaluating information;

Jayne Benkendorf, my special friend and business associate who has spent years studying nutrition and how to improve health, for her valuable help in proofreading and clarifying information;

Dale Hammond, professor of chemistry at Brigham Young University at Hawaii, for answering almost endless questions about enzymes and their role in healing the body.

Table of Contents

FOOD COMBINING
Better Health — The Natural Way

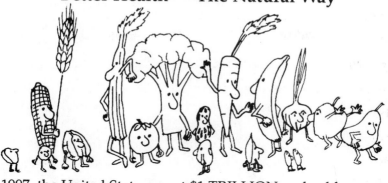

In 1997, the United States spent $1 TRILLION on health care—just in hospitals and doctors' offices. That's $3,000 for every man, woman and child. We also spent staggering amounts on nutritional supplements in health food stores. So, are Americans the healthiest people on earth? In comparing the United States to 227 other countries, it ranked **29th** in infant mortality and **46th** in life expectancy!! That means that people in 28-45 countries spend far less on health care, have far better health and live longer lives than Americans, according to Dr. Ted Morter, author of *Dynamic Health.*

The USDA food pyramid recommends 6-11 servings of grain per day, and most of those servings are eaten in the form of processed grains (pasta, pizza and breads). Yet, the majority of nutrients necessary for good health and prevention of cancer and virtually all other diseases come from fresh fruits and vegetables, NOT from processed grains.

Do you feel *healthy*, or do you have chronic aches and pains and frequent illnesses that require prescription or other drugs? Would you like to feel **better**? Could you use more **energy** without relying on caffeine or other stimulants? Do you worry about getting **cancer, diabetes, arthritis, or other degenerative diseases**?

Whether you are just beginning to use wholesome foods (or maybe still thinking about it??), or are already using them on a daily basis, this handbook will show you how to **combine** and **prepare them properly** to get the most from your meals. It will reveal the secrets of good nutrition and give you the keys to eliminating disease so you can enjoy BETTER HEALTH ...THE *NATURAL WAY*.

WATER

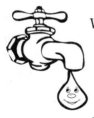

Water is essential to life. Seventy percent of our bodies are composed of water, so they REQUIRE water to function *every* day. The radiator in your car won't run on coke, tea or coffee; neither will your body. Water isn't just something you should *drink*. Water is vital to the proper functioning of your body. People who have been deprived of water have died within a few days, while others have survived for weeks and sometimes months without food because they had an adequate supply of water.

Water brings valuable oxygen and nutrients into our cells. It carries away carbon dioxide and other waste products, and cushions and protects important body organs such as the brain, spinal cord, and lungs. Water helps to keep the body temperature normal. Nearly three-fourths of the body is made up of water. Some of that water is used up or eliminated (in urine, sweat, etc.) and should be replaced regularly. You lose 8 to 12 cups of water each day. Drinking less than that amount can damage the body.

KIDNEY AND LIVER FUNCTION

Water is essential to proper kidney function. When the kidneys are inefficient, the liver must take over, reducing available energy and efficiency. According to Marilyn Diamond, author of *Fitonics For Life*, sixty million Americans are overweight (twice as many over the last hundred years). This is astounding in view of the fact that the average consumption of calories has been reduced by 10%.

The liver already has a big job to do in metabolizing stored fat into readily available energy, so when the liver takes over for the kidneys, it is forced to *metabolize less fat*. **Less fat is burned and more fat remains stored.** When insufficient water is consumed each day, it is almost impossible to lose weight.

FLUID RETENTION

Fluid retention is your body's way of conserving water when supplies are low. The cure is not in the temporary "quick fix" of pills that get rid of water (diuretics). Just give your body what it needs—**more water**. Excess salt may be to blame, but drinking more water will dilute the concentration.

CONSTIPATION

Water is also essential in ridding the body of waste and avoiding or relieving constipation. Toxins increase during weight loss. If you eat too many foods with low water content and fail to drink adequate water, the colon quickly becomes clogged and constipation results. This causes even more toxins to be released into the body. Normal bowel function usually returns when water is increased.

HOW MUCH WATER IS ENOUGH?

Most doctors recommend that people drink at least 2 quarts of water per day. More is needed in hot weather and when vigorously exercising. For overweight people, drink one additional glass for every 25 pounds of excess weight. This can be accomplished by drinking a quart in the morning, a glass with each meal or snack, and anytime in between, with the remainder in the early evening. Cool water is easier to drink in large quantities than ice water. If you're eating a normal American diet and waiting until you're really thirsty to take a drink of water, you're already dehydrated.

WATER WITH MEALS

Many people teach that drinking lots of water with a meal dilutes the digestive juices, slows down digestion, speeds up putrefaction, and causes foods to be passed through the body without giving up their valuable nutrients. According to Drs. Remington, Fisher and Parent, as stated in *How To Lower Your Fat Thermostat*, "unless you have had part of your stomach removed," there is no reason why you can't have a small glass of water with each meal.

HIGH-WATER-CONTENT FOODS

You won't be thirsty for as much water if you eat high-water-content foods that require lots of chewing, like raw vegetables, sprouts or juicy fruits. If you want to have bread, have a veggie sandwich made with toasted whole grain bread or a bagel and pile it up with lots of cucumbers, leaf lettuce, tomatoes, sprouts, peppers, grated carrots or cabbage, etc. (Chewing foods thoroughly allows starches to be broken down and mixed with enzymes found in the saliva, so *chew, chew, chew.*)

In addition to having high water content, "live" foods (raw, as close to fresh-picked as possible, not wrinkled or wilted) contain essential enzymes that will provide more energy than cooked foods.

When you eat at least 5 servings per day each of juicy water-packed raw fruits and vegetables, you will not be as thirsty as when you eat breads, pasta, crackers, and salty foods.

When you've been eating juicy foods for a few months, start to listen for your body's signals. Are you really thirsty? You may not need more than an occasional glass of water after drinking a quart in the morning. Six cups (total) per day should still be the absolute *minimum* unless you are very active or trying to lose weight.

PURE WATER

Regular tap water is usually loaded with chlorine and other harmful inorganics, often making it taste too nasty to drink! Purchase bottled water (tastes good but is not always pure), or a system designed to filter *and* purify. I prefer a system that uses reverse osmosis along with a carbon filter designed to eliminate impurities larger than .2 to .5 microns.

To purify water that has been stored for a while, or that may be contaminated (from rivers and streams, or unsafe water supplies in foreign countries), I add 3-5 drops of grapefruit seed extract to each glass of water, 20-30 drops to each gallon. This all-in-one anti-bacterial product is also an excellent household cleaner for toothbrushes, vegetable/fruit or meat/poultry wash, sterilizing dishes and utensils, cutting boards and any other "germy" surface.

Healthcare professionals worldwide use this liquid concentrate as nutritional support for individuals with certain health concerns, such as sore throats, colds, and flu. It is excellent as a dental rinse, throat gargle, ear rinse, nasal spray, facial cleanser and scalp treat-ment. This product is a MUST for every home to help eliminate bacteria the *natural* way. For information, call 1-888-232-6706.

FLAVORED WATERS

If you just can't face drinking large amounts of plain water, try this recipe for flavored water from my friend Jayne Benkendorf (author of *The Food Bible*). To 3 cups of pure water, add 1 T. fresh lemon juice and 1 cup red or purple grape juice (use only brands that are 100% juice). This just slightly flavors the water while quenching thirst. I like to drink this at any time during the day, but especial-ly when I need to drink a LOT of water.

To summarize, the purpose of drinking water is not to wash down the food we eat. So WHY do we need water?

1- Water is the BEST thirst-quencher
2- Water takes valuable nutrients to the right parts of the body
3- Water transports toxins OUT of the body

If you've been working or exercising hard and you're VERY thirsty at mealtime, drink a large glass of water 15 minutes before your meal and eat high-water-content foods.

HIGH-WATER-CONTENT FOODS

The high water content of your body requires the water lost each day to be replaced. Besides drinking water, you should also be eating high-water-content foods - whole fruits and vegetables and sprouted grains, legumes, seeds and nuts. Eat most raw for a "healthy" supply of enzymes and vitamin C. Only about one-fourth of your diet should be from concentrated foods such as cooked breads, grains, meat, dairy products, legumes, nuts and seeds.

High-Water-Content Food Diet

TYPE OF FOOD	NUMBER OF SERVINGS	TOTAL VOLUME
Nuts & Seeds	Optional	1/4 c. (2 oz.)
Legumes	1-2	1/2 to 1 c. cooked or sprouted beans, peas or lentils
Fruits	3-5	1 1/2 to 2 1/2 c.
Vegetables	4-6	2 to 3 c. dense or 4 to 6 c. leafy
Whole Grains*	4-6	2 to 3 cups cooked or sprouted (1 slice bread = 1 serving)

If using meat or dairy products in your diet, reduce the number of servings of grains, or eat them sprouted.

Note: Sprouting turns concentrated foods (nuts, seeds, legumes, grains) into high-water-content foods and provides enzymes that change starches into easy-to-digest sugars.

The American Institute for Cancer Research (AICR) agrees that the majority of our diet should be plant-based, rich in a variety of vegetables and fruits, legumes and minimally processed starchy staple foods.

The American Dietetic Association's *Daily Food Guide* suggests that vegetarians make sure to include "1 cup of dark green vegetables daily to help meet iron requirements." For those not using milk or dairy products, the *Food Guide* suggests using soy milk.

RAW FOODS

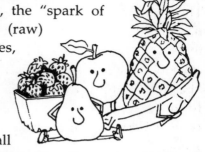

ENZYMES are protein molecules, the "spark of life" present in all UNCOOKED (raw) fruits, vegetables, grains, legumes, nuts, seeds and even meats! Every chemical action and reaction in the body requires an enzyme. The nutrients in foods are "locked" and cannot be broken down into small enough particles to be utilized by the body unless a special "key" is provided—**enzymes**! Besides aiding in the digestion of food, enzymes *repair* cells within the body. The body makes a specific enzyme to repair the heart, one to repair the kidneys, and so on.

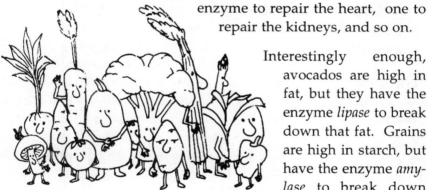

Interestingly enough, avocados are high in fat, but they have the enzyme *lipase* to break down that fat. Grains are high in starch, but have the enzyme *amylase* to break down starch. *Protease* enzymes break down protein and *cellulase* enzymes break down fiber. Enzymes also break down fats, starches, proteins and fibers already present in the body.

Only a small amount of each enzyme molecule is required to break down these foods. The remaining portion is then sent to the "enzyme bank" until it is called upon to break down foods that don't have their own active enzymes, such as cooked foods. (Raw foods carrying their own enzymes are digested more quickly and are less likely to ferment in the stomach and end up as toxic waste than foods for which the body must go to the "bank" and search for the right enzyme.)

ENZYMES ARE DESTROYED AT 130 DEGREES F.

Americans eat MOST of their food cooked. Some don't eat ANY raw fruits and vegetables on a daily basis. Enzymes begin to die at 118°F and are completely destroyed at 130°F. Cooked foods lack these absolutely *essential* molecules. When a body isn't FED enzymes, it cannot do a good job of MAKING enzymes or of BREAKING DOWN foods into usable molecules.

This may sound like a simple problem, but what happens when the body can no longer make sufficient enzymes? Indigestion is first on the list. We are a nation plagued with indigestion, but that is only a minor part of our ailments. Cooking foods (except lightly steaming or stir-frying) kills the very enzymes all foods NEED in order to be broken down small enough to pass through the minute pores of the intestines into the blood stream.

When we eat fresh foods that are past their prime, or are overcooked, cell REPAIR cannot take place. Imbalances are created and the body begins to weaken. The immune system doesn't have what it needs to fight illness. We set ourselves up for all degenerative diseases, including cancer and arthritis. In a talk by Dr. Joel Robbins, noted biochemist, the U.S. Surgeon General is quoted as saying that "70% of all deaths related to stroke, heart disease and cancer are *preventable through diet.*" **The body IS capable of making repairs to damaged cells to lessen or eliminate disease. Recent research shows that whole, raw foods, complete with enzymes, are the key.**

What's the best way to start getting a good supply of enzymes? Make sure to eat "live" fresh fruits or vegetables at every meal and for snacks. Include lots of fresh, leafy or crunchy sprouts. They're cheap, easy to grow and require no special preparation. See *Natural Meals In Minutes*, Section 2, for a complete guide to buying, storing and sprouting seeds of all kinds.

WHOLE FOODS

WHOLE foods are just that - whole! If an apple has been peeled, it's not WHOLE. If wheat has had the outer hull taken off, the wheat germ and the wheat bran removed, and bleached to produce white flour to make the melt-in-your mouth cakes, cookies, pastries, fluffy white pancakes, or boxed instant breakfast cereals, it's not WHOLE! If brown rice has been stripped of its fiber to produce white rice that makes such quick and easy side dishes, it's not WHOLE.

WHY ARE WHOLE FOODS IMPORTANT?

Americans have the most abundant food supply in the world, but we are far from being the healthiest people in the world. Why? It's what we DO to our foods that makes the difference. We eat the highest percentage of cooked, processed, refined foods of all "civilized" countries. These processed foods are in every grocery store and nearly every home. They are certainly abundant in every school cafeteria! They form the basis for every meal. What are they? Sugared cereals, white bread, pretzels, chips, crackers, cookies, muffins, cakes, candies, white pasta, soda pop, juice drinks, sugary jams and jellies, prepared dinners and "fast" foods. Let's see, is there anything "fun" to eat that I forgot? If so, add it to the list!

These foods provide less fiber, fewer nutrients, and more quick-burning calories. They cause malnutrition (even in affluent societies), lack of energy, sluggish digestion and elimination, and upset the delicate balance of the immune system. *What's left to eat?* Believe it or not, there are hundreds of delicious, wholesome foods waiting for you that will fill you up, slim you down, give you energy, take away your cravings, and *put you on the road toward better health.*

HOW IMPORTANT IS A HEALTHY IMMUNE SYSTEM?

A malfunctioning immune system allows the following to occur:

- Weight abnormalities - too much or too little fat. The immune system regulates how we absorb, digest and store food, how efficiently we convert nutrients to energy, and whether we burn fat for energy or store it as excess weight
- Allergies and sensitivities to foods, chemicals, fabrics, dust and pollens, etc.
- Auto-immune diseases — arthritis, lupus, Crohn's, AIDS
- Cancers
- Common cold, flu, infections, etc.

What CAUSES a weakened immune system? Stress, food additives (including sugar), chemicals, drugs (including alcohol and tobacco) and hidden food allergies are the major culprits in immune system malfunction. Other causes include: starvation or liquid diets; skipped meals; over-consumption of cooked foods; excess acid-forming foods such as meats, all dairy products and cooked grains; and all refined foods (white flour, breads, desserts).

Good nutrition isn't just some weird "health nut" soapbox topic. During the last 20 years, research has proven that good nutrition DOES rebuild the immune system. "Isn't it ironic," says Dr. Dean Ornish, "that it's considered 'radical' to exercise, relax and eat a heart-healthy diet." Good nutrition is *essential* to your better health. The choice is up to you. *How much better do you want to look and feel?*

Is immunity something that can be bought? Yes, if you start by buying the freshest foods available (or grow them yourself). The second step is to prepare them correctly. (Other factors are also important, like learning to eliminate negative stress, practicing positive thinking, and getting adequate sleep and exercise. Most people, however, already know they need to work on these things.)

IMMUNITY-STRENGTHENING FOODS

Category	Recommended Foods
Grains	Whole grain cereals, breads, muffins; brown or wild rice; oats; barley; rye; corn; millet; bulgur or cracked wheat; specialty grains such as teff, millet, spelt, kamut, triticale, amaranth, quinoa, etc.
Seeds	Raw sesame, pumpkin, sunflower, flaxseed.
Nuts	All fresh, raw (preferably soaked).
Vegetables	Mostly raw, lightly steamed or stir fried. Include leafy green vegetables daily.
Legumes	All beans, peas and lentils, sprouted and/or cooked.
Sprouts	All kinds, most eaten raw, especially wheat, oats, barley, quinoa, adzuki, mung, soy, pea, lentil, garbanzo, pumpkin, sunflower, clover, buckwheat and alfalfa.
Fruits	All fresh (most eaten raw); frozen (unsweetened); low-heat process dried fruits (unsulphured).
Proteins	Reduce consumption of meats and replace with small quantities of gluten, tofu, TVP, and plant proteins such as nuts, seeds, grains, legumes, preferably sprouted.
Oils	Cold-pressed oils; olive, sunflower, canola.
Beverages	Fresh fruit and vegetable juices; bottled or frozen juices (100% juice only - no sugar sweetened juices)

ENERGY

Next in importance to *healing* the body, these immunity-strengthening foods are our BEST sources of energy for *fueling* the body. What IS energy? Calories! What is the best source of calories? Complex carbohydrates. If you think calories and carbohydrates are the ENEMY, read on.

Most people cut *calories* to lose weight. But calories don't count!!! Yes, the body needs calories, but if you must count something, count *nutrients*. Many people still gain weight on 1000 calories per day. They complain of no energy and poor health. Others successfully lose weight, increase energy and improve their health on 1000 calories per day. Why?

The body doesn't just need *calories.* If it did, we would all enjoy excellent health while eating pure white sugar. EVERY body needs the *nutrient-dense calories* found in wholesome, unrefined fresh fruits, vegetables, nuts, seeds, grains, and legumes.

What about the 2000 calorie per day USDA Food Pyramid Recommendation? The fact that most Americans are overweight shows that it's not working! Most people eating 2000 calories per day consume too many unnecessary and even harmful calories in the form of *refined sugar* found in soft drinks and candies, as well as *refined carbohydrates* in the form of pasta, most breads, cakes, cookies, donuts, etc.

If you consume enough **unrefined** complex carbohydrates (all foods from the plant kingdom) to fill you up each day (with 4-5 servings per day eaten raw), your body will be fueled by a steady supply of calories that are chock full of essential nutrients to build and heal the body.

Will ANY unrefined complex carbohydrates do? No, in order for the body to heal, or to maintain health, it has to be slightly alkaline and no one can tell you **exactly** what you should eat to stay in that alkaline state. I can only provide guidelines, because EVERY body is different. You can experiment with how many calories (nutrients) you need, how much raw food you need, and how much processed food you can handle. It's your body, so it has to be your choice.

Dr. M. Ted Morter, Jr., author of *Dynamic Health,* has done extensive research in the area of achieving the proper acid/alkaline balance to enable the body to heal and rebuild cells. He, too, recommends that *at least* 70% of our diet be composed of high-water-content foods, because these foods leave an alkaline ash when processed by the body. Unsprouted grains and all animal or dairy products leave an acid ash, but the body can usually handle a diet of about 30% acid foods. In his book *Your Health, Your Choice,* Dr. Morter wrote that "the food you ate yesterday was broken down, parts of it were assimilated, used or stored, and other parts were discarded. The first urine of the morning contains much of the material that has been processed out while you were sleeping. While you sleep, your body is busy repairing, restoring, and replenishing cells, tissue, and organs. At the same time, it prepares unusable residue, toxins, and other extraneous parts of food for elimination." Testing the urine using his guidelines will enable you to "read" your body and develop the plan that's right for you.

I was surprised that my very "nutritious," mostly-vegetarian diet, was actually very *acid.* I learned that I ate far too many *cooked grains* in an effort to follow the USDA recommendations.

For more information on learning how to tell if the foods you choose are right for YOUR body, call Dr. Morter at 1-800-281-4450.

GOOD CALORIES = LONG-LASTING ENERGY

Some calories actually damage the body, increase hunger, and cause overeating and weight gain. These calories are found in all refined foods (white breads and pastas, white sugars, artificial sweeteners). Because these foods are refined to remove the fiber that normally slows down digestion, the body is able to convert them quickly into energy. This quick energy causes the blood sugar to rise rapidly, followed by a corresponding sharp rise in insulin, which the body releases to regulate the blood sugar. The rise in insulin works so well that it then forces the blood sugar levels to "crash," thereby making you feel hungry again. If you then eat MORE refined food, the process is started all over again. All this is damaging enough, but when insulin levels are high, *the body burns fewer calories and converts MORE calories into fat!* Also, the immune system ceases to function when insulin levels are high.

Dr. Richard N. Podell, in his book *The G-Index Diet* has created an index showing the glycemic response, or effect on blood sugar, for a large number of foods. Foods are divided into categories of *highly desirable, moderately desirable,* and *less desirable.* Refined foods and most grains cause a quick rise in blood sugar, are high on the Glycemic Index, and are always in the less desirable category. These foods should be eaten only occasionally, or combined with fresh, raw vegetables to prevent a rise in blood sugar. Foods eaten RAW (especially when sprouted) are highly desirable and always low on the G-Index.

Remember that enzymes are responsible for breaking down foods, and even if you're eating wholesome high-fiber foods, if they are ALL cooked, they can't be utilized properly. To help keep insulin levels low, digestion normal, and the body well nourished, eat lots of raw food meals, or at least *eat raw foods at the start of every cooked food meal to supply the body with enzymes to process what follows.*

HOW TO GET THE MOST ENERGY FROM YOUR MEALS

1- **Whole grains** are supposed to be **good** for you. So why not just eat 4-6 slices of 100% whole wheat bread each day? Whole wheat bread is a better choice than white bread, but is still processed much too quickly by the body. A better choice would be to make or buy "hearty" breads that require *chewing*, like those containing bits and pieces of seeds and cracked or sprout ed grains, and to serve them with lots of raw or lightly steamed non-starchy **vegetables**. An even better choice would be to eat most grains whole or cracked. The best way to eat grains is sprouted, with some eaten raw.

2- Eat most **fruits** raw and without sweeteners.

3- Eat some raw **vegetables each day, especially dark-colored ones and leafy greens**.

4- Sprout **legumes** (all beans, peas and lentils) to eliminate gas and to increase availability of nutrients. Sprouted beans cook in only 15 minutes.

TO SUMMARIZE: Most good calories come from fresh fruits and vegetables because these foods are alkaline, loaded with valuable nutrients, and full of FIBER. Raw or lightly steamed foods are the lowest on the glycemic index, are the ONLY foods with essential enzymes and are therefore the least likely to cause an insulin response.

Are you wondering if you can ever again indulge in a sweet treat, pizza or french fries? SURE! Feeding your body MOST of the time from *good calories* allows your metabolism to work much more efficiently, so the occasional indulgences are less likely to cause major problems. And, as you begin to **feel** better, you're less likely to make poor food choices.

FIBER

Whole, natural, high-fiber foods can be friend or foe. When switching from refined to whole foods all at once, foods are rushed through the body too quickly for the body to absorb nutrients. This can cause diarrhea, especially when adding the *insoluble* fiber of grains that travel quickly through the body, cleansing and scouring. Adding the *soluble* fiber of legumes that travel slowly, absorbing water and adding bulk to the stools, solves the problem!

THE FIBER–CHOLESTEROL CONNECTION

Fiber, most broadly, is the portion of plant foods our bodies can't digest. It comes in two basic categories — insoluble and soluble. Insoluble fibers, which *don't* dissolve in water, are the more obviously "fibrous" of the two. These include the woody or structural parts of plants, such as fruit and vegetable skins and the bran coating around wheat and corn kernels. They pass through the digestive tract largely unchanged and speed the passage of whatever else comes along for the ride.

Soluble fibers, which *do* dissolve in water, are found in abundance in beans, oats, barley, broccoli, prunes, apples, and citrus fruits. They have the consistency of a gel and tend to slow the passage of material through the digestive tract. The process of refining foods removes much of the insoluble fiber — hence the widespread NEED for bran and other fiber supplements and laxatives. Research has shown that cultures that eat only whole foods have no need for extra fiber, nor do those cultures suffer any of the health problems caused from the lack of adequate fiber.

HOW MUCH FIBER IS ENOUGH?

British physician Denis Burkitt found that the rural Africans he studied ate some 50 to 150 grams of fiber a day. Americans, by contrast, typically consume about 20 grams. It is generally accepted by many researchers today that we should double or triple our fiber intake (mainly soluble fibers, eaten as unrefined foods) and cut our fat consumption at least by one half. To increase soluble fiber intake, we could eat 3 c. of oatmeal per day! Or, how about 1 1/2 c. of oat bran, or 3 standard doses of Metamucil, Fiberall, or other bulk laxatives? *One cup of beans provides the same amount of fiber,* is much more pleasant to eat and can be served in an endless variety of meals, such as bean dip, bean burritos, or creamy soups.

Since beans are one of the richest sources of fiber and an excellent source of protein with almost no fat, they are one of the best sources of soluble fiber. They also provide a rich source of essential minerals, especially when sprouted.

Increasing fiber foods has the effect of lowering cholesterol - in some cases dramatically. Also important, however, is cutting back on cholesterol-rich foods. This can easily be accomplished by replacing meats with legumes and grains.

FIBER IN GLUTEN-FREE DIETS (CELIACS)
Until recently, it was believed that celiacs should avoid fiber, specifically grains. Now, with patience, even those with damaged digestive systems can use white rice flour and finely ground bean flour, gradually working up to using brown rice flour.

Those with extreme sensitivities should grind their own flours or check with the manufacturer of commercially ground flours to be sure they are milled in a wheat-, oat-, barley-, and rye-free environment. Since beans do not have the scouring effect of grains, they are generally well tolerated.

FATS

During infancy and childhood, normal brain development requires fats. Fats provide energy and support growth. As the most concentrated source of energy available to the body, one would think we needed LOTS of fat, but after the age of two years, the body actually requires very little fat. For nearly 15 years, we've been told to cut down on saturated fats, most of which come from animal products. We are now eating 10% less fat. Why, then, are we as a nation fatter than EVER?

1- Butter has been replaced by margarine that is supposed to be better for us because it contains vegetable oil. What we're not told is that the vegetable oil used to make margarine is *hydrogenated*. Hydrogenated oils (heated and refined vegetable oils) are found in nearly every product on the grocery shelves, and are even WORSE for the body than the saturated fats found in butter!

2- Manufacturers discovered they could make "sweet nothings" without fat if they increased the sugar. People reasoned that if a container of ice cream were fat-free, then the whole thing was a legal indulgence. Not so! Research shows that fat is made by the body from excess calories - from too much fat, too much sugar, or just too much food! Excess fat creates more fat. Excess **sugar** creates more fat. Excess calories of ANY kind are used to create more fat.

3- With so many "time-saving labor devices," we have eliminated much of our physical work. We have become much more sedentary, burning fewer calories **and** less fat.

4- Many health-conscious people assumed that since saturated fats are bad, ALL fats must be bad. They stopped eating the naturally high in fat foods like cold-pressed oils, raw nuts and seeds, olives and avocados, that actually help **reduce** the blood levels of "bad cholesterol."

IS THERE SUCH A THING AS A GOOD FAT?

Recent research shows that the body does need some fat, but only "good" fats. You've all heard of "good" cholesterol and "bad" cholesterol. The body needs some "good" fats in the form of *essential fatty acids* to protect us from the devastating diseases like heart disease, cancer and stroke.

Essential fatty acids are found in fish oils and in unrefined vegetable oils such as cold-pressed (unheated, uncooked) flaxseed oil, olive oil, grape seed oil, primrose oil, and in many natural foods...the very foods we've eliminated in our efforts to *cut the fat!*

Research scientists worldwide are rediscovering the benefits of good fats in fighting disease and lowering cholesterol. In addition, studies have shown that fats help slow down digestion of foods that would normally be high on the glycemic index. For instance, bread with high-fat avocado slices would digest better and allow the body to maintain more stable blood sugar levels than bread eaten alone.

Adding the right amount of good fats can actually help aid weight loss by adjusting metabolism naturally, increasing the body's ability to burn excess calories. The good fats even help eliminate the bad fats from our cells and tissues. Flaxseed oil is one of the best-tasting sources of essential fatty acids. It is virtually tasteless when added to smoothies or mixed with maple syrup for pancake topping. Olive oil is touted as the best cooking oil. I like sunflower oil for baking and in place of butter on popcorn.

Research done by the National Cancer Institute found flax to have an anticancer effect—without the side effects of traditional cancer treatments. Flaxseed has been called "heart smart" because of its ability to lubricate and relax blood vessels, and to help clear clogged arteries.

The good fats found in flax combat infection and allergies by boosting the immune system. They have been shown to be helpful in improving memory, behavior, and mental ability. In a study done on school children fed bread products containing flax, attendance and behavior even improved! Flax has also been helpful in relieving inflammation and arthritis pain by balancing the hormones that aggravate these conditions. People with eczema (my grandchildren included) have also found relief by including flax seeds and flax oil in their diets.

HOW MUCH FAT IS NEEDED?

A National Academy of Sciences' anti-cancer report warns that Americans are eating too much meat, too much protein (especially animal protein) and too much fat - over 40% of total calories. The report recommends we reduce all dietary fats to 30%, while other doctors and researchers now insist total fat intake must be cut to 5-10% in order for the body to heal and prevent disease. If you're scratching your head, wondering how all these %%% relate to the food you eat every day, let me paint a graphic picture.

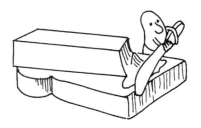

On an average 2000 calorie diet, 40% of calories eaten as FAT each day would be equivalent to buttering a slice of bread with nearly 1 full STICK of butter! When eaten one handful of chips at a time, one hamburger at a time, one french fry at a time, one slice of pizza at a time, or one cookie or candy bar at a time, it doesn't seem possible to consume that much fat in a day. But it is, and we do, because most fats are *hidden*. Where? Most corn or potato chips contain about 1 gram of fat per chip. Tostitos baked chips have only 1 gram per 20 chips! When eaten with a no-fat salsa or my 5-Minute Black Bean Dip, I can't tell much difference. I would much rather eat 20 chips rather than only ONE. Wouldn't you? I would also rather make bread without fat so I can spread it with a little butter.

Cutting back to 30% of calories eaten as fat would only cut your chunk of butter to about 2/3 of a cube, and 10% of calories would equal 1 1/2 T. of butter.

If your goal is to lower cholesterol and promote healing from or prevention of ALL diseases, use polyunsaturated fats (from corn, soybean, safflower and sunflower oils), or monounsaturated fats (from vegetables and nut oils such as olive, flax, peanut, and canola), and stay away from saturated fats and all products with trans-fatty acids (all hydrogenated or partially hydrogenated oils).

Cutting down on fat isn't as hard as it seems. Nearly all recipes calling for oil can be altered by simply leaving it out (salad dressings, soups and dips), or adding a mashed fruit such as bananas, applesauce, or prunes (all breads and baked goods). If I eliminate the fats that are non-essential, I can thoroughly *enjoy* the essential ones, like olives and avocado in a salad, almonds and flax oil in a smoothie, or a small portion of butter or almond butter on bread.

FLAXSEEDS TO THE RESCUE!
These "good fat" seeds can be coarsely ground and sprinkled over cereals, rice, pasta, vegetables, and fruits. Ground seeds mixed with ground raw almonds and raisins or dates make an excellent power-packed "energy bar." Flaxseeds can be added to all breads and baked goods.

A tablespoon or two per day of the seed or oil has produce significant health benefits in numerous studies. It can be added to smoothies, salad dressings, sandwich fillings, pancake syrups, granola, and many more things. The oil should *always* be used raw.

PROTEIN

Dr. James Balch, author of *Prescription for Nutritional Healing*, explains that the body manufactures a *different* type of protein to form each different body component such as hair, bones, muscles, ligaments, organs, nails and vital body fluids. The body can use ONLY amino acids to manufacture these proteins. There are eight essential amino acids that must be obtained from the diet. The approximately 20 other commonly known amino acids are produced by the liver.

EXCESS PROTEIN CONSUMPTION

Most Americans consume 200% to 400% more protein than needed, resulting in serious health problems. Some of the health abnormalities related to excessive animal protein consumption are: heart disease, arteriosclerosis, premature aging, mental illness, mineral imbalances (causing severe calcium and magnesium deficiencies, as well as deficiencies in vitamins B6 and B3). Sources include the U. S. Army Medical Research and Nutrition Laboratory, Dr. Lennart Krook, and Dr. Uri Nikolayev, as well as doctors from Holland and Denmark.

The National Academy of Science urges us to replace the fattier animal protein with low-fat plant protein, such as whole grains, dried beans, peas, lentils, soybeans and soy products.

According to leading authorities on heart disease, Dr. Dean Ornish; pediatrics, Dr. Lendon Smith; and many others, the body obtains all the amino acids it needs to build protein from plant sources. It is, however, still possible for even strict vegetarians to get too much protein in their diet.

HOW MUCH PROTEIN IS ENOUGH?

Research has shown that any excess protein (from ANY source) is converted into carbohydrates; then, if not burned as energy, it is converted to fat, just as if you ate a huge banana split. Excess protein also puts undue stress on the kidneys and liver, so it is best to rely on foods from the plant kingdom to supply the body's needs and to monitor closely the protein intake from ALL sources. When using concentrated sources of protein, like milk, cheese, tofu, gluten, TVP and protein powders, it is still possible to eat too much protein, regardless of the source.

Mother's milk is only about 1 1/2% protein. On this small amount, a baby is able to double its birth weight several times within a few short months. If all that growing and developing takes only a tiny amount of protein, why are we told we *need* so much more?

George Beinhorn, in *Bike World Magazine*, states: "The United States Government's own 70-gram recommendation was established on the basis of research that clearly showed 30 grams to be *completely adequate*. The extra 40 grams were labeled a 'margin of safety.' Though one Food and Nutrition board member reported that the real reason behind the high figure was that the board feared a 'public outcry' over the 30 gram figure."

Eating too much protein at one sitting forces the body to try to *process* it all at once. Your car's fuel tank can only take so much gasoline. Any excess you try to put in is wasted. If you overfill your body's fuel tank with too much protein (or too much of *any* fuel), the excess fuel creates harmful toxins that the body must try to process and eliminate.

The body works best with a constant supply of high-quality fuel, so spread out your protein consumption during the day.

HOW MUCH FOOD DOES IT TAKE TO EQUAL 30 GRAMS OF PROTEIN?

Eating 4 servings per day of grains and 1 serving of legumes provides about 22 grams of good quality protein. A typical day's food choices might include the following: 1 c. brown rice (5g), 1/2 c. black beans (8g), 1 pita pocket (6g), and 1/2 c. cracked wheat pilaf (3g). Other fruits and vegetables contain small amounts of protein, usually 1/2g to 1g per serving (potatoes and dark green vegetables provide 3-5g per serving!), making it very easy to get enough protein without adding protein powders or animal proteins.

A little protein powder (1 T = 12g) in a smoothie or a small amount of meat (1 ounce = 6g) or eggs (1 = 6g) eaten as a salad garnish or as an occasional side dish would be acceptable if you cut down on your servings of grain or legumes. But remember, the body needs fiber to move foods quickly through the digestive tract, and it doesn't get ANY fiber from animal proteins.

ANIMAL PROTEIN IS A LOW-QUALITY FUEL

The proteins that make up the human body are NOT obtained directly from the foods we eat. The body must first break down foods into individual amino acids, the "building blocks" of protein. Animal protein, especially beef, the American "protein of choice," is considered a low-quality fuel for humans because there are very strong bonds holding the amino acids together. This requires that the body expend about half as much energy as that food supplies just to try to liberate the amino acids. The human body is not good at breaking these strong bonds, so the mostly-intact chain of amino acids then becomes toxic because it passes too slowly through the body.

According to Dr. Norman Walker, author of *Diet and Salad Suggestions*, this process creates a vast amount of uric acid that is absorbed by the muscles where it crystallizes and causes rheumatism, neuritis, sciatica, etc. Thousands of analyses of urine show that without exception, the uric acid present in the urine of meat eaters was far less than what should be eliminated, indicating that the muscles were absorbing from 5 to 10 times what the body **should** eliminate through the kidneys.

On the other hand, foods from the plant kingdom are easy for the body to use because they contain **loosely bound** amino acids that are easy for the body to separate and recombine as protein. When you eat a good supply of enzyme-rich plant foods, it doesn't TAKE energy for the body to MAKE energy from plant proteins. The nutrients from plant foods are quickly and easily broken down, then efficiently transported through the body. These are the "high octane" fuels the body needs to run smoothly and efficiently.

COMPLETE AND INCOMPLETE PROTEINS
Plant protein comes from three main classes of foods: legumes (beans, peas and lentils), nuts and seeds, and grains. Proteins from plant sources are "incomplete proteins," because one or more of the eight essential amino acids is missing or in short supply (with the exception of soybeans).

Legumes must be combined with another protein source, from another class of foods, such as seeds or grains (or animal products). They are born mixers as well as meat extenders. They can be mixed with grains or meats to stretch your dollar and improve nutrition.

A meal containing legumes and seeds; legumes and grains; or seeds and grains provides all the amino acids needed to supply protein for health and growth. These incomplete proteins can even be eaten as much as 24 hours apart and still combine properly because the body stores the excess amino acids in reserve to be used on an "as needed" basis. When cells need repair, the body can't wait for food to be eaten. It relies on its reserves to supply the necessary amino acids in the right quantities to form the kind of protein necessary for the part of the body needing repair.

FOOD COMBINING FOR PROTEIN COMPLEMENTATION

This makes meal preparation much less complex, and allows us to consume meals combined for proper digestion and let the body do the work of figuring out what it needs from this meal...and that meal...and the next meal...and so on.

As long as we don't "gum up the works" with processed fats, refined flours and sugars, we can count on getting all the protein we need to run our "fine machine" just by following the recommended servings shown in our Natural Food Pyramid.

According to Dr. Lendon Smith, "Eliminating, or drastically reducing meat and dairy products creates a large void in the diet of most Americans. The benefits of using beans on a daily basis have recently been promoted because studies show beans help to reduce cholesterol while providing excellent nutrition. When combined with nuts, seeds or grains, they form a complete high-fiber vegetable protein.

"A three-ounce steak will provide 350 calories and only about 15 grams of usable protein. One and one-fourth cups of cooked beans will provide the same number of calories and yet deliver 50% *more* usable protein. And, since beans are only 2-3% fat, you have a virtually fat-free source of protein, with NO cholesterol.

"By using beans ground to a flour in all your baked goods, you not only create a perfect protein, you also add valuable B vitamins, carbohydrates and iron. Creamy soups, sauces and gravies to rival canned or packaged brands are thickened with bean flour and are made without any fat or dairy products. Busy cooks will be happy to know that these soups and sauces cook in only 3 minutes. They're almost instant, and much *more* nutritious and much *less* expensive than those available from the supermarket."

COMPLETE PLANT PROTEINS
Gluten (GLOOtun) is made from whole wheat flour and contains the 8 amino acids necessary to make up protein. However, the amino acid lysine in most wheat is low. Adding bean flour in the gluten-making process will add the necessary lysine.

Tofu (TOEfoo) is a complete protein and is made by curdling the milk of soybeans with an acid. It is a concentrated protein with a bland flavor that can be seasoned or eaten plain. It makes excellent creamy smoothies and ice cream.

TVP, also a complete protein, is a commercial meat substitute made from soybeans that have been processed at very high temperatures. It is not as easy to digest as gluten and tofu.

COMBINING PLANTS FOR PROTEIN

Properly combining foods from the plant kingdom produces a high quality low-fat protein that is rich in fiber, vitamins and minerals...with NO cholesterol.

High-protein plant foods are divided into three groups, as shown on the chart at the right. Each category is usually low in one or more amino acids and needs to be combined with foods of another category that are high in that amino acid. The body will then break down these foods into amino acids and store them for up to 24 hours. If foods from corresponding categories are not eaten within that time, the stored amino acids are discarded as waste.

Eating a wide variety of foods ensures that your body will have the right "raw materials" to manufacture a good supply of protein.

EXAMPLES OF FOODS IN EACH CATEGORY

LEGUMES: *Anasazi Beans, Adzuki Beans, Black Lentils, Black Beans, Blackeyed Peas, Fava Beans, Garbanzo Beans, Green Lentils, Green Peas, Kidney Beans, Lima Beans, Mung Beans, Navy Beans, Peanuts, Pink Beans, Pinto Beans, Red Beans, Red Lentils, Scarlet Runner Beans, Small White Beans, Soybeans, Tofu and Soy Products, Yellow Peas*

NUTS & SEEDS: *Almonds, Brazil Nuts, Cashews, Filberts, Pecans, Flaxseeds, Pumpkin Seeds, Sesame Seeds, Sunflower Seeds, Walnuts*

GRAINS: *Amaranth, Barley, Buckwheat, Corn, Millet, Oats, Quinoa, Rice, Rye, Spelt, Teff, Triticale, Wheat*

Note: Dark green vegetables are a good source of iron and protein, as well as many other essential vitamins and minerals. For best nutrition, eat a wide variety of fruits and vegetables every day. OR, sprout foods from the above categories.

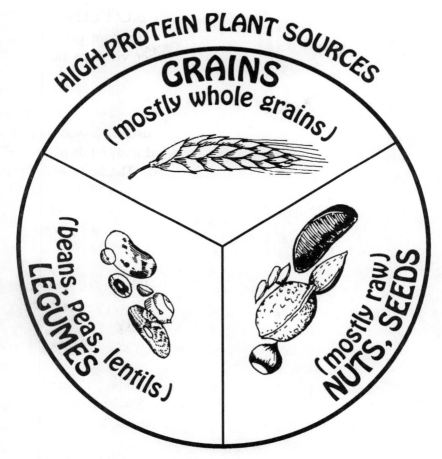

HIGH-PROTEIN PLANT SOURCES

GRAINS
(mostly whole grains)

LEGUMES
(beans, peas, lentils)

NUTS, SEEDS
(mostly raw)

COMPARE THE COST

Not only are plant proteins more easily digested and utilized by the body, they are *much* less expensive. When served as a source of protein, beans cost less than 10¢ per serving, compared to commercial cheeses at 40¢ per serving and meats at a minimum of 75¢ per serving! (Idaho Pea and Lentil Commission)

WHEAT PROTEIN FOR LOW COST MEALS

Gluten is a mixture of proteins found in wheat and to a smaller degree, in oats, barley and other cereal grains. It helps make dough rise. When separated from the starch and bran in wheat, gluten is an excellent meat substitute. It is high in protein with NO cholesterol and only a trace of fat in each serving. It is much more easily digested than meat, very easy to make into "fake meats," and very inexpensive. LeArta Moulton, in *The Amazing Wheat Book*, gives the following figures:

> 12 c. whole wheat flour makes 4 c. raw gluten which bakes into 9 c. ground gluten which is equivalent to 3 lbs. cooked hamburger! The wheat flour costs only 56¢ and yields:
>
>
> 512 gluten cubes (1/2"x1/2")
> 150 meatballs
> 20 steak slices (4"x1/2")
>

What's the current cost in *your* store for 3 lbs. of extra lean hamburger, or extra-lean steaks? (Note: Even if you can *afford* extra-lean hamburger, can you afford the 232 grams of fat, 93 grams of saturated fat, or the 940 milligrams of cholesterol, without ANY fiber, in 3 lbs. of meat? Compare that to only 27 grams of fat, 4 grams of saturated fat, NO cholesterol, and 36 grams of fiber in 3 lbs. of gluten.)

WHAT ABOUT FIBER FROM PROTEIN FOODS?

Foods from the animal kingdom do not contain ANY fiber. Fiber is present only in plants. With most Americans consuming large amounts of animal protein, white bread, white pasta, white rice, and refined cereals, it's no wonder we suffer from constipation, colon cancer, diverticulitis, colitis, and a host of other fiber-related illnesses. Look at the following chart to see how much fiber can be obtained from ordinary foods. Note: Most foods from the plant kingdom are VERY low in fat. Most high-protein foods from the animal kingdom are very high in fat.

PLANT FOOD	PROTEIN	FAT	FIBER
1 slice whole wheat bread	3g	1g	3g
1 c. asparagus	5g	1g	2g
1/2 c. cooked barley	8g	Tr	5g
1 spear broccoli	5g	1g	3g
1 c. corn	5g	1g	4g
1 c. ground gluten	31g	2g	4g
1 c. peas	5g	1g	7g
1 potato	5g	Tr	4g
1 whole wheat pita	6g	1g	3g
1 c. frozen spinach	6g	Tr	8g
1 c. regular oatmeal	6g	2g	4g
1 c. whole grain macaroni	7g	1g	3g
1 c. brown rice	5g	1g	3g
1 waffle	7g	4g	2g
1 c. beans, peas, lentils	15g	1g	7g
1" slice regular tofu	9g	5g	1g
1" slice Mori-Nu lite tofu	9g	2g	1g

MEAT	PROTEIN	FAT	FIBER
3 oz. sirloin	23g	15g	0g
3 oz. beef roast	19g	26g	0g
3 oz. ground beef	21g	16g	0g
3 oz. pork chop	24g	19g	0g
2 slices bologna	7g	16g	0g
3 oz. chicken breast, skinless	28g	3g	0g

Plant proteins win hands down in my kitchen! Does that mean I never eat meat? No, but it does mean that I don't rely on meat as a source of protein. I use meat **sparingly,** as a garnish, rather than making it the main ingredient in my meals. We typically use one pound of chicken breasts to season 12 cups of taco mix made with beans, rice, onions, and taco seasoning (homemade, of course!), at a cost of about 40¢ per cup. Compare that to $2 per cup using commercial taco mix and extra lean hamburger. Now that's what I call really s t r e t c h i n g your food dollars!

CALORIES

HOW MANY CALORIES?

Since the foods we eat are supposed to provide us with energy, vitamins, minerals and other essential nutrients, how many calories a day does it take to get what we need? The typical American diet provides adequate (often far more than adequate) calories, but does it provide enough nutrients? (The USRDA for calcium has increased from 800 milligrams per day to 1,000 because studies have shown that most people are calcium deficient, despite the increase in calcium-rich dairy products.)

USDA RECOMMENDATIONS

According to the National Academy of Sciences, the recommended daily caloric intake of 2,700 for men and 2,000 for women are designed for physically ACTIVE adults, ages 23-50. (These figures are based on the consumption of the typical American diet consisting of excessive fats, refined carbohydrates and sugars.)

According to Drs. Remington, Fisher, and Parent, authors of *How To Lower Your Fat Thermostat*, the average male eats about 3,000 calories; the average female eats about 2,000 calories, with about 40% of those calories coming from fats (down from almost 50% with the recent advent of "fat-free" commercial products) and sugars (mostly refined). Refined or processed fats and sugars have almost *no* nutrients. Consider this study that analyzed the number of calories consumed vs. the nutrients obtained:

	MALES	FEMALES
Total Calories Consumed	3000	2000
Fat calories	1200-1500	800-1000
Sugar calories	600	400
Total fat and sugar calories	1800-2100	1200-1400
Remaining Calories containing vitamins and minerals	*900-1200*	*600-800*

From this example, it doesn't take much figuring to determine that the huge number of calories consumed as fats and sugars (mostly from fried foods and desserts) leaves very little room for *wholesome* foods that contain vitamins and minerals.

Where are we supposed to get these important nutrients? They certainly don't come from "enriched" products. If someone borrowed $1 from you and returned 15¢, would you feel "enriched?" This is what the food manufacturers do when they refine out wholesome nutrients and fiber (real food) and replace it with a small amount of artificial nutrients (fake food).

Can a typical male get *enough* vitamins and minerals from the 900-1200 calories' worth of food; or a female from 600-800 calories? Not according to any of *my* textbooks! Based on these figures, it's no wonder we have such cravings for food and tend to overeat! Our bodies are literally *starving* but not for more of the same food—just for REAL food.

REALISTIC RECOMMENDATIONS

A more realistic caloric figure to supply essential vitamins and minerals is 1500 calories for men and 1000 for women. These nutrients are from REAL food - fruits, vegetables, whole grains and legumes. Adding small amounts of raw nuts, seeds, honey, *good* fat and occasional fish or poultry provides an additional 300-600 calories from fat, carbohydrates and protein.

To increase calories further, add extra servings of low in fat starchy complex carbohydrates in the form of whole grains, whole grain pasta, potatoes, corn and legumes. Following these guidelines, the caloric intake for men should be in the range of 2,000 to 2,500; 1,300 to 1,800 for women. The following chart gives a breakdown of which foods should supply what percentage of daily calories:

HEALTH-PROMOTING DIETARY RECOMMENDATIONS

FOOD CATEGORY	PERCENT OF TOTAL CALORIES
Fats	10-20%
Proteins	10-15 %
Complex Carbohydrates	60-85%
Refined Carbohydrates	0% or Very Few

DETERMINING THE RIGHT NUMBER OF CALORIES FOR YOUR BODY

While the above recommendations give you the guideline for choosing a balanced diet from wholesome foods, the real key to determining the right number of *calories* for your particular needs is whether you feel satisfied after a nutritious meal and whether that feeling lasts until snack or meal time.

Consuming fewer "bad" fats and sugars may take a few days for your body to get used to, but you will quickly feel how much it enjoys live, whole foods and the energy they contain (once you get over sugar "withdrawal" symptoms).

WHY NOT JUST EAT FEWER CALORIES?

Some people manage to stay thin while eating almost exclusively artificially sweetened drinks, candy, and fat-free desserts. Fresh fruits, veggies, whole grains and legumes are NOT in their vocabulary OR their pantry. They eat very small quantities of food to keep their calories low and still be able to eat what they want.

Over the years, these people (many of them young) have suffered from various ailments, with the symptoms eased by a ready supply of prescription drugs. Without exception, the people I know have aged quickly, have NO energy, and most have gained large amounts of weight, even while consuming only 400 calories a day!

The body has a built-in survival mechanism that adjusts to the foods (or non-foods) we eat. Some bodies can survive on starvation diets for a period of years, but that doesn't mean there aren't changes going on in the body!

According to Drs. Remington, Fisher and Parent, "A decrease in food intake below that needed to maintain the body weight at set-point (the body's 'normal' weight) results in an increased appetite and a decrease in energy wasting (the rate at which the body uses energy).

"Of course, if a person is *really* starving, this mechanism is truly important, allowing the person to adapt to the next episode of starvation by having an even larger amount of fat stores, as well as having a body designed to protect those fat stores. The problem is, the body's survival mechanism can't distinguish between starvation and dieting. These adaptive responses... may lie dormant for long periods and cause no particular problem until triggered by a period of unwise dietary efforts.

"The weight-regulating mechanism then recognizes that the food intake has decreased and that the body weight is starting to fall. In an attempt to defend the weight, the body starts conserving energy and stimulates the appetite. The weight loss soon stops *even if the dieter can resist the stronger urges to eat.* If the person gives up and goes back to his normal caloric intake, the body weight may increase because it now [has adapted to fewer calories by using] less energy. If the dieter wants to continue losing, he must *further* reduce his food intake.... Even then, weight loss will eventually stop." When the dieter gives in to hunger and increases calories, "weight will most likely increase *again* to its previous normal level, since the body has become so much more efficient." (Sounds like a clear case of "danged if you do and danged if you don't" to me!)

What's the answer? Changing the *quality* of calories is simple compared to staying on a starvation diet, and much easier to stick with than most weight loss programs. The body responds well to high-quality fuel in the form of wholesome foods because these foods do more than FEED the body; they *nourish* the body. Within a matter of months, the "setpoint" can be reset to a new lower level.

WHAT ABOUT STUBBORN SETPOINTS?
Because of thyroid and other glandular malfunctions, it is possible for a person trying to lose weight to eat a low-calorie "healthy" diet and still not lose weight. In working with many people of this type, I have found that eating mostly enzyme-rich raw foods and few, if any, cooked foods is the solution. Raw foods provide far more energy and are much more easily digested, leaving the body free to burn stored fats. Including lots of sprouted grains, nuts, seeds, beans, peas and lentils ensures a good supply of calories and protein plus the freshest vitamins and minerals on earth.

Combine sprouts with raw vegetables for an endless variety of "whole meal salads." Try sprouted garbanzo, sunflower and quinoa with shredded jicima, broccoli stems, and banana or butternut squash. Top with toasted pumpkin or sunflower seeds, a few slices of avocado, and a "good-4-u" dressing.

EXERCISE

EXERCISE??? IN A FOOD COMBINING HANDBOOK?

Moderate exercise makes EVERYTHING work better, including the body's ability to process foods more efficiently. Moderate exercise helps stimulate digestion as well as elimination. A person who exercises regularly is less likely to be troubled with constipation OR diarrhea.

When we breathe, we take in oxygen, which combines with glucose to break the chemical bonds of hydrogen and oxygen, allowing energy to be released. When we work or exercise hard enough to require EXTRA oxygen, extra energy is released. When I open the glass door on my fireplace, more air is drawn from the room, across the fire and up the chimney. The fire burns brighter, the flames leap higher, and the wood burns faster, using up oxygen and quickly requiring more. The same thing happens when we exercise hard enough to increase breathing and heart rate.

EXERCISE TO OPERATE AT PEAK EFFICIENCY

Most of us don't work hard enough physically to obtain the amount of exercise our bodies need to build and maintain muscles. Muscles burn fat for energy, so if you lose muscle through lack of activity, extreme dieting, or even illness, your body will have less capacity to operate at peak efficiency. In addition, the right kind and amount of exercise is an important factor in total mental well-being, allowing your brain to operate more effectively. I don't know about you, but I can use a clear mind and a more effective brain *any* day of the week!

EXERCISE TO DEAL WITH STRESS MORE EFFECTIVELY

We all experience physical and emotional stress throughout our lives. The ease with which we handle this stress depends to a great extent on our physical condition. Regular exercise helps us deal with these situations in a more calm and efficient manner. The increased oxygen to the brain from regular exercise helps us think more clearly, quickly, and logically. Many have experienced a greater level of creativity when they exercise regularly. It seems plain that exercise and increased activity throughout the day need to be an important part of our lives.

As an extra bonus, you will have more strength and energy to do the things you didn't get done during the valuable time you gave up to exercise! Losing excess fat (while toning up muscles in the process) will add years to your life, and a lot more zip to your years!!

HOW MUCH EXERCISE IS TOO MUCH?
Many studies have shown that 30 minutes of exercise per day is completely adequate. It doesn't even need to be all at the same time! Exercising longer is OK, but only if you *enjoy* it. In one study, participants engaging in at least one hour of intense aerobic exercise per day lived only about 2 years longer than those who were physically active, but did no *regular* exercise—the same amount of time it took to DO the exercise!!

LEARN TO BURN MORE ENERGY
Use up more energy every day and you'll need less "exercise." While you may not have the energy to do anything extra at first, after a few weeks, you'll notice a spring in your step and energy you didn't know was possible. This is a sign that fat energy is being released and used as fuel.

So, BURN that energy as you sprint to the mailbox or from one end of the house to the other; push, pull, tug, lift - exert yourself a little more each day; park your car farther from the store or work;

carry your own groceries, even if it takes two trips; use the stairs rather than the elevator or escalator; dance, even if it's by yourself in your own home; do leg lifts and arm circles while waiting for a phone to ring or when you're on hold; join a walking or hiking club and enjoy the scenery while you walk off your fat; plant a garden and work in it often.

Doing things to save steps or energy may be the most *efficient*, but we're trying to get RID of fat, not conserve it! Why conserve steps doing housework or gardening, then spend an hour exercising? If you're sitting in front of the television or the computer so long that you get dusted along with the furniture, you can bet you're storing up fat by the minute.

WHAT TYPE OF EXERCISE IS BEST?

For best results, choose some form of weight-bearing exercise, such as walking, stair-climbing, cross-country skiing, treadmill, trampoline, etc. Exercise bikes, rowing machines and swimming are fine if you have a physical problem which keeps you from standing, but results will not show as quickly. Some pools have exercise boots and dumbbells with fins to increase resistance. These are used in shallow water as well as deep water. This equipment does a good job of raising the heart rate and is a great form of exercise.

Walking can be done every day, but if you're doing any other type of exercise, give your muscles a break and wait at least 48 hours before repeating that exercise. You may want to walk one day and cross-country ski or jump on a mini-trampoline the next. Remember, though, you'll burn the most fat, give your muscles a rest and have a chance to exercise a different area of your body if you choose an exercise that involves *both* arms and legs.

FOODS FOR ENERGY

Real food is **full** of real energy, and energy heals! Many people have experienced healing from life-threatening diseases simply by eating wholesome foods and allowing the body's immune system to function as it was designed.

Doris Grant and Jean Joice, in their book *Food Combining for Health*, discuss the findings of Dr. William Howard Hay, born in 1866. Dr. Hay turned to the field of Natural Health only after he had been diagnosed with several diseases in his early forties, and was given only a short time to live. Within three months, his symptoms were gone! He felt better, lost his excess weight, and launched on a new era in healing where he proved the folly of "fussing with the end results of a condition instead of attempting to remove the cause."

Over and over, as the years passed, Hay proved repeatedly through the results obtained in his practice that "the body is merely a composite of what goes into it daily in the form of food and drink." Modest man that he was, Hay never claimed to have invented anything new. He simply had learned to feed the body what it needed to *allow* natural healing forces to be able to do the job the Creator intended.

THE IMPORTANCE OF CORRECTLY COMBINING FOODS

High-protein foods and foods eaten in the wrong combinations create an "acid" condition in the body. It is this condition that fuels multi-billion dollar profits by antacid manufacturers. Have you ever heard an antacid commercial that told you to take responsibility for what you do TO your body and to stop eating so much or to stop eating so many different kinds of foods at one meal? No! The common solution to acidity is to just take more or stronger antacids! What happened to old-fashioned responsibility? Whose job IS it to keep you healthy? It's YOUR job. You can CHOOSE to have better health.

WHAT FOODS CREATE ACID?

Eating proteins (eggs, milk, fish, chicken, beef, or even tofu!) at the same meal as starchy carbohydrates (pasta, potatoes, rice, bread, or beans) is the #1 cause of acid indigestion. These foods are eaten together at nearly every meal in America. Why do they create acid?

Each different type of food requires a different enzyme for digestion, and a different amount of time for processing before that particular food leaves the stomach. Proteins are broken down by the hydrochloric acid found in the stomach. Starches begin to be broken down by the alkaline digestive juice, ptyalin, found in saliva. The two conditions of acid and alkaline cannot exist together; one or the other will be at least partially neutralized. What happens then? There will most likely be too *much* acid for the starches to be digested, and too *little* acid for the proteins to be digested. When food can't be digested properly, it begins to spoil, resulting in the acid indigestion that creates the need for antacids!

So, you ask, if you can't have chicken and rice, beef on a burger, or eggs over hash browns, what IS there to eat? You can still eat the same foods, but you'll feel better if you change the way you combine them. You can eat a meal of chicken strips or chopped, boiled eggs in a chef salad; veggieburgers on a bun, with a fresh, green salad and steamed veggies; pasta with vegetable sauce, lots of fresh vegetables and fresh bread, or chili *(without the meat)*, corn bread and fresh veggies.

Does this mean you can't eat chicken-noodle soup; a little Parmesan cheese on your pasta; or rice protein powder in a smoothie? No, this principle doesn't apply when SMALL amounts of one food group are combined with a large amount from another. If you are eating sufficient raw foods, there *should* be enough enzymes present in your food and stored in your enzyme bank to properly digest meals with the slightly less than perfect combination of a *little* protein with a *lot* of starch.

The typical American meal consists of large quantities of animal protein and starchy vegetables, like potatoes, peas, and carrots. Few, if any, high-water-content vegetables are eaten, and most are cooked to death. The Chinese typically have very small quantities of meat with their rice, and an abundance of tender-crunchy vegetables. Rather than "garnishing" our plates with salads and vegetables, we should be *filling* our plates with them, and adding the proteins and starches as the garnish.

WHAT DOES ALL THIS HAVE TO DO WITH ENERGY?
First of all, most people spend at *least* half of their energy digesting food. If your body is busy dealing with the crisis of digestion *every* time you eat, you're left with less energy than you really need to make it through the day.

It's no wonder so many people turn to caffeine drinks, alcohol and other stimulants to be able to keep up with their daily responsibilities. Wouldn't you love to have enough energy to make it through the day without any stimulants?

REACH FOR AN ENZYME RATHER THAN ROLAIDS®
In the section on *enzymes*, it was stated that energy is supplied and healing takes place when raw foods are eaten. Dr. Sydney Crackower in *Two M.D.'s And A Pharmacist Ask, "Are You Getting It 5 Times A Day?"* says that you can easily create the "perfect meal" at any time of the day just by adding enzyme-rich foods. Dr. James Balch states that sprouts are the richest source of enzymes. By adding sprouts, you can create a meal filled with energy, *and* the ability to take care of its own digestion, even when eating a meal of mostly cooked foods.

The four categories of enzymes found in the body and in raw foods (especially sprouts) each have a very different specific function:

- Lipase breaks down fat
- Protease breaks down protein
- Cellulase breaks down cellulose (fiber)
- Amylase breaks down starch

Eating raw foods daily helps supply digestive enzymes to prevent the body from having to use its own enzymes to break down fat in the food you eat. Enzymes also help break down any excess body fat that's just "hangin' around." Raw foods containing lipase are the ones that have naturally-occurring "good" fat like avocados, nuts, and cold-pressed vegetable oils. Eat small amounts often.

Many people have been taught *never* to combine fruits and vegetables at the same meal. Adding fresh fruit to a vegetable salad, or juicing carrots, peaches and pears together would have been considered digestive suicide only a few short years ago. New enzyme research, however, shows that RAW fruits and vegetables perform perfectly together.

Sprouting nuts, seeds, legumes and grains activates essential enzymes and makes them as easy to digest as raw fruits and vegetables, even if they are then cooked. **Soaked** almonds, even though they are high in protein, digest well even when combined with a starchy food such as bananas.

What about the warning never to combine starchy grains with fruits? Forty years ago, my mother started serving sprouted wheat with banana slices at demonstrations to teach people how to eat simple, basic foods. Seminar participants noticed that this pleasant combination failed to produce the normal stomach upset they would normally have had from combining fruits and grains, such as bread with jam, cereal with fruit and/or sugar, etc.

The reason is now crystal clear: RAW foods have no combining limitations! In addition, sprouting converts the starch in grains to a sugar and breaks down the sugars and proteins in legumes. (Personally, knowing that I *could* add bean sprouts to a fruit salad doesn't fill me with anticipation, so I will still continue to eat my sprouted beans separately or add them to sandwiches or vegetable salads.)

A whole wheat pita, spread with almond butter and stuffed with clover sprouts, is a fantastic meal! Even though the whole grain bread and the almonds are cooked, rendering their enzymes inactive, the fresh sprouts do a great job of ensuring that the starches and fats will be broken down so they can be properly utilized without digestive chaos!

Is this all too **WEIRD** for you? Consider the option of living *without* enzymes to heal. Why would anyone *want* to be stuck with an immune system that can't fight off disease; a mind that can't think clearly or process information effectively; a body that must have drugs in order to relax muscles, or to be calm, peppy, thin, digest food, relieve constipation, or stop diarrhea; a heart that can no longer pump sufficient blood; cancer that destroys body parts and most often life itself; kidneys that fail to purify the blood or a liver that can no longer filter body wastes and manufacture amino acids to create protein?

These problems are considered *normal*, and it would be *weird* not to be plagued by them. That's my kind of weird, and I promise that you'll learn to like weird as much as I do when you see the results of following these few, simple guidelines.

If you do, however, you will always be in the minority, as evidenced by a recent survey, where nearly half of the respondents ate NO fruits and vegetables that day. Only about a fourth had three or more vegetables and slightly more than a fourth had two or more fruits. Less than ten percent of the people surveyed actually ate the recommended 5 fruits and veggies. In similar studies, NO respondents ate their fruits and veggies RAW so they had good enzyme activity! Is it any wonder that we're a nation plagued with disease when we are surrounded by an abundance of the very foods to CURE disease?

ENZYME SUPPLEMENTS
You can purchase enzymes in pill and liquid form that aid in digestion, but there is no perfect substitute for REAL foods, especially raw foods. An enzyme supplement should contain at least three of the essential enzymes: protease, amylase, and lipase, to digest protein, starch, and fat. The missing enzyme, cellulase, breaks down fiber, and since we traditionally eat such *small* amounts of fiber, this is the one enzyme manufacturers often leave out.

The best and only complete, *active* enzyme supplement source (with all the essential vitamins and minerals) I know of is Juice Plus+, with 17 different fruits, vegetables and grains.

Many doctors are now prescribing this product for their patients rather than traditional medicines, because they now recognize that *it is the active enzymes that will heal their patients*—not the drugs that have been relied on for so many years. They recognize that drugs only **suppress** symptoms. Enzymes heal the body and **eliminate** the symptoms.

These physicians, along with many thousands who belong to or are affiliated with the Physicians Committee for Responsible Medicine (PCRM), and the American Institute for Cancer Research (AICR), are finally able to watch true healing take place as the body receives the essential raw materials to heal *itself* as it was designed to do.

RECIPES

The heart-healthy recipes in this section are family favorites—low in fat, high in fiber, protein, and other valuable nutrients—and made from the best foods on earth! While these recipes do not contain meat, I am not a vegetarian. I don't live where I can buy meat that is properly fed and handled, so most often, I choose not to eat it. In times of famine or extreme hunger, I would use meat on a regular basis, but for now, I have plenty of other options.

If you choose to add meat to these recipes, you do not need to make any special adjustments; add small quantities of lean meat to Grain and Garden Burgers, Soups, Salads, etc. Or, serve it on the side as a garnish.

This section of recipes has been compiled to give you a "taste" of the fantastic meals you'll find in the following cookbooks (see ordering information in the back of this book):

Natural Meals In Minutes - *Bingham*
Country Beans - *Bingham*
1-2-3 Smoothies - *Bingham*
Quick Wholesome Foods video - *Bingham, Moulton*
The Amazing Wheat Book - *Moulton*
Cookin' With Home Storage - *Tate*

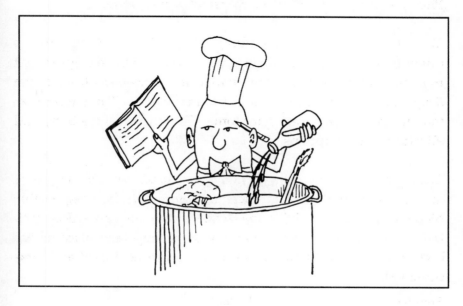

Natural Meals In Minutes *(Bingham)*

This book uses grains, legumes, sprouts, dry milk powder, fresh fruits and vegetables to create 30-minute meals your family will love! Nearly 300 recipes in three sections. Valuable sprouting information and techniques.

GRAIN AND GARDEN BURGERS

2 c. cooked brown rice	1/8 t. black pepper
2 egg whites or 1 egg	2 T. red lentil flour
1/4 c. grated onion	3/4 t. salt

Mix well. Place 1/4 c. of mixture in a skillet coated with cooking spray. Shape and flatten with a spatula. Cover pan and cook over medium-low heat until browned on both sides.

Serve plain or topped with white bean gravy, barbecue sauce, or cheese. OR, serve on a bun with all the fixin's. Serves 4.

SUPER EASY SUN SALAD

2 c. 3-day sprouted sunflower seeds
1 T. lemon juice   *1 t. olive or sunflower oil*

Mix all ingredients, adding salt to taste, and serve plain or on a bed of lettuce or clover sprouts. Serves 4.

CREAMY 3-MINUTE PUDDING

2 c. hot water	1 egg or 2 egg whites
1 T. butter (opt.)	1 t. vanilla
1/3 c. honey	3 T. cornstarch
1/3 c. dry milk powder	1/4 t. salt
1/8 t. lemon extract	4 c. fresh fruit

Put all ingredients except fruit in blender and blend until smooth. Pour into medium saucepan and bring to a boil over medium heat. When thickened, reduce heat to low and cook an additional 1 minute. Cool and pour over fruit such as fresh or frozen strawberries and fresh bananas.

Country Beans *(Bingham)*

Learn to use legumes (and sprouted legumes) in recipes that will change the way YOU use beans! Nearly 400 recipes, most gluten-free. Over 115 bean flour recipes. Make a meal of these recipes by adding fresh, *raw or lightly steamed* non-starchy vegetables.

5-MINUTE REFRIED BEANS

2 1/2 c. water
1/2 to 3/4 t. salt
tiny pinch garlic powder (opt.)

3/4 c. pinto or black bean flour
1/4 t. cumin
1/2 t. chili powder

Bring water to a boil in a small saucepan. Whisk in dry ingredients. Cook, while stirring, over medium heat for 1 minute, until mixture thickens. Reduce heat to low, cover pan and cook 4 minutes. Add 1/2 c. Picante sauce, if desired. Mixture thickens as it cools and will stay thick even after heating.

3-MINUTE "CREAM OF CHICKEN" SOUP

6 c. boiling water
1 c. fine white bean flour

2 T. chicken or vegetable bouillon
1 c. diced chicken pieces (opt.)

In a medium saucepan over medium heat, whisk bean flour into boiling water and add base. Stir and cook 3 minutes. Blend for 1 minute. Add chicken, if used. Serves 3-4.

SUPER CORN CHIPS

1/4 c. fine corn flour
1 t. fine pea flour
1/2 t. dry taco seasoning mix

1/2 c. water
1/8 to 1/4 t. salt

Blend just until smooth. Spoon batter, 1 t. at a time, into circles on a lightly oiled baking sheet. (If too much oil is used, crackers will not get crisp.) Tilt tray to spread circles very thin. Bake at 350° for 8 minutes, or until edges curl and center is set. Turn over; bake another 2-5 minutes until golden and crisp.

1-2-3 Smoothies *(Bingham)*

123 Quick Frosty Drinks — Delicious AND Nutritious! Healthy fruit-filled drinks that can be used at any time of the day. Learn sneaky ways to add nutritious ingredients into smoothies even finicky eaters love!

PEACH PERFECTION
1/3 c. Welch's 100% White Grape Peach concentrate
1/2 c. water   *1 c. frozen peaches, cubed*
1/2 c. rice milk   *1 frozen banana*
4 small ice cubes   *Opt. 1/2 t. acidophilus powder*

Place rice milk (or any other type of milk) and all remaining ingredients in blender in order given. Blend until smooth and creamy. Makes 3 cups. Serves 2-3.

SWEET RASPBERRY CREME
1/2 c. Welch's 100% White Grape Raspberry juice concentrate
3/4 c. low-fat soy milk   *1 t. vanilla extract*
2 ripe pears   *1 frozen banana*
6 small ice cubes   *Opt. 1/2 T. rice protein powder*

If using protein powder, blend with milk until smooth, about 1 minute. Add remaining ingredients and blend until thick and creamy. Makes 4 1/2 cups. Serves 3-4.

Sauces, Seasonings & Natural Meals *(Bingham)*

Over 200 recipes using whole foods to create healthy sauces, seasonings, and delicious, nutritious meals. Most are gluten-free, dairy free.

ONION SOUP MIX (Lipton substitute)
1/2 c. powdered chicken bouillon *1/16 tsp. white pepper*
1 c. dried, minced onion   *1/4 t. black pepper*
1/2 c. onion powder   *1/4 c. parsley flakes*
4 T. cornstarch   *1/8 t. basil*
1 T. chives

Note: 12 bouillon cubes makes 1/4 c. powder. Combine all ingredients and store in an air-tight container. Use 1/4 c. mix in place of one Lipton Onion Soup packet.

Quick Wholesome Foods *(Bingham/Moulton)*

This 65-minute video features new techniques and information for making your Food Storage into unbelievably delicious meals the whole family will love! Whole Wheat Breads, Gluten, Wheat dishes for every meal of the day, 3-minute Cheeses from powdered milk, and user-friendly Beans.

SEAFOOD SALAD

2 c. cooked cracked wheat

1/2 c. catsup

1 diced tomato

One 6 1/2 oz. can drained tuna (opt.)

1/2 c. mayonnaise (low-fat)

1/2 c. each diced green onions, green peppers, celery

Using cooled cracked wheat, mix all ingredients well. Serve on a bed of lettuce and sprouts, in pita pockets, or on toasted whole wheat bread. Serves 6.

SECRET SOUP

4 c. boiling water

2 1/2 T. chicken bouillon or soup base

3 c. sprouted white beans

Cook beans in water 20 minutes. Blend beans with water to cover for 3 minutes, or until very creamy and smooth. Add 2 cups cooked, diced potatoes and carrots. Serves 4-6.

PIÑA COLADA SPREAD

4 T. cream cheese

2 T. shredded coconut

1/2 t. lemon juice

2 T. honey

1/2 t. vanilla

Mix well and spread on crackers or beat until fluffy and use as a frosting for cookies, cakes or muffins. Makes 1/2 cup.

SAUSAGE SEASONING FOR GLUTEN (see recipe on next pg.)

1 T. white pepper

1 T. black pepper

2 T. salt

1 t. sage

1 t. nutmeg

1 t. savory

1/2 t. garlic powder

Mix, store in air-tight container. Makes 1/3 cup. For 2 c. seasoned gluten, add 1 T. mix, 2 eggs, 2 T. wheat flour, and 2 T. olive oil. Form into patties or balls. Bake at 350°F for 20 min.

The Amazing Wheat Book (Moulton)

Fast, easy recipes for wheat meats, seasoning mixes, perfect breads, crackers and desserts.

RAW GLUTEN — Using Vital Wheat Gluten flour
2 c. gluten flour   *1/3 c. soy flour*

Mix well and add the following:
2 c. hot water   *3 T. seasoning of your choice*
                     (onion soup, taco, bouillon, etc.)

Stir liquid into flours (takes only about 10 stirs). Place in a vegetable steamer and steam, covered, until firm, about 20-30 minutes. Grind with electric food processor or hand meat grinder.

WHEAT CHIPS
1 c. whole wheat flour   *2 c. water*

Mix well and season to taste with *one* of the following:
1/2 t. ea. onion and garlic salt *1 T. seasoning of your choice*
1 t. salt or vegetable salt   *(onion, taco, barbecue, etc.)*
3-4 T. parmesan cheese

Stir ingredients together to form a thin batter. Pour mixture into squirt bottle, as shown in video, and squirt onto non-stick sprayed cookie sheet in potato chip shapes. Bake at 350° for 10-15 minutes or until crisp. Turn chips over during baking if middle is not cooking as fast as outside. Note: Thinner batter = more crisp chips.

Cookin' With Home Storage (Tate)

Over 700 food storage recipes, including pioneer recipes, home remedies, natural beauty and personal care, and survival tips.

WHOLE WHEAT PANCAKE MASTER MIX
24 c. whole wheat flour   *4 T. salt*
8 T. baking powder   *4 c. dry milk powder*
2 1/4 c. powdered eggs

Mix and store in cool, dry place. To use, stir together just until moistened: 2 c. dry pancake mix, 2 1/2 c. water and 2 T. oil. Cook on medium hot lightly greased griddle, turning when edges are set.

INFORMATION

Whether you're a seasoned cook or a novice in the kitchen, you're sure to discover some totally new information in this section that will help you make low in fat, high in flavor, easy-to-digest meals—faster than you ever thought possible!

In this section of valuable information you'll learn how to:
- *Crack and grind wheat and other grains and beans for the freshest breads, cereals and wholesome meals on earth.*
- *Use wheat and bean flours to make gluten, an easy-to-digest complete high-protein meat substitute.*
- *Sprout grains, beans, nuts and seeds for "garden-fresh" produce during any season of the year.*
- *Combine plant foods to form complete protein meals.*
- *Combine plant foods properly for best digestion.*
- *Provide complete nutrition every day using the Natural Food Pyramid.*

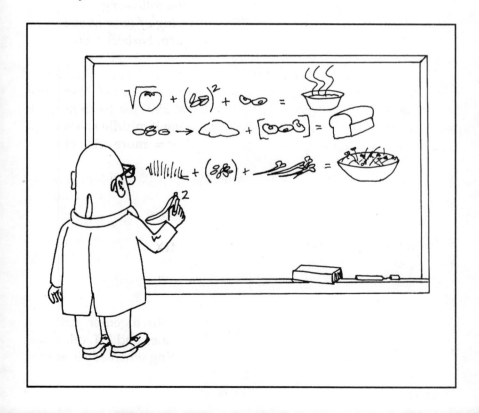

CRACKING AND MILLING WHOLE GRAINS AND BEANS

Modern equipment for the kitchen has revolutionized the use of whole grains and legumes. They can be ground to a fine flour using a hand grinder for small quantities, or electric mills for larger quantities.

WHY MILL YOUR OWN WHEAT AND LEGUMES?
Fresh flours are far superior in taste as well as nutrition to commercially ground and forever-stored flours purchased from grocery stores and most food co-ops. As soon as the outer hull of a grain or legume is cracked, the nutrient content begins to decline, due to oxidation. This leads to rancidity, which has been shown to be cancer-causing. Flours should be used within one month or stored in an air-tight container in the refrigerator or freezer and used within 3-6 months.

Other grains, such as millet, barley, oats, rye, etc., can be milled and added to any recipe calling for wheat flour for increased nutrition and to vary flavors. Adding legume flour to grains supplies essential amino acids to produce a complete protein.

There are several good mills on the market, electric and manual, that produce a fine flour from whole grains. There's no better smell than breads, pancakes, or muffins from freshly ground whole grain flours. Gluten, made by adding water to wheat flour, then separating off the bran and starch tastes best when made using freshly milled flours.

WHICH MILL IS BEST?
My electric favorites are the K-TEC and the GrainMaster Whisper Mill because they are guaranteed to grind all grains, beans, peas,

and lentils. Other companies say their mills *will* grind beans, but won't put their guarantee in writing. For emergencies, my favorite hand mill for grinding grains, peas and lentils (whole corn and large beans must first be cracked), because of its small size and relatively small price, is the Back To Basics mill.

Larger hand mills and other electric mills are available from preparedness stores like Country Store & Kitchen Specialties (360-256-9131), Preparedness Plus (801-226-4188), and Walton Feed (1-800-847-0465). Check out Lehman's Catalog (330-857-1111) for many other hand mills that will grind ALL grains and beans, with prices ranging from $45 to $565. Ask about #C-17B + #C-7A (abt. $230).

HOW TO MILL GRAINS AND LEGUMES
Sort grains or legumes, checking for broken seeds, pieces of dirt, or small rocks, and pour into hopper of your mill. I like to mill outside, or in my garage. To mill inside, place mill in the kitchen sink and cover it with towels to capture most of the fine dust from grinding. Set mill to grind on medium-fine. The resulting flour should be as fine as the wheat flour you use in baking breads, cookies, etc.

Turn the mill on. Larger beans will need to be stirred where they go into the grinding chamber (with the handle of a spoon) so they will not get stuck. When grinding more than 12 cups of grains or 4 cups of legumes, make sure to change the sponge filter, "flicking" out flour buildup, or using a clean replacement filter.

Legumes that have absorbed excess moisture, or ones with a high oil content, like garbanzo and soy, will cause caking on electric mill parts. Thoroughly brush away flour residue from all parts of the mill after each use. If you have a lot of buildup, grind a cup of dry grain to help clean out internal parts.

After milling, I clean my mill with a small 2" paint brush to clean off any excess flour. To avoid weevils and mold, make sure to clean and store your mill properly.

CRACKING GRAINS

Whole wheat takes about 1 hour to cook. Cracked wheat brought to a boil, then covered and removed from the heat, takes only 15 minutes. It is easier to chew, easier to hide in ground meats and sandwich fillings, and easier to pass off as meat when made into "burgers." It also makes excellent breakfast cereals as well as salads.

WHAT GRAINS CAN BE CRACKED?

All grains CAN be cracked. The ones I use most are wheat, oats, corn and brown rice. These make excellent breakfast cereals and meatless patties.

HOW TO CRACK GRAINS

Most electric mills will not crack grains or legumes. I use a small electric seed or coffee mill (Cuisinart, Proctor-Silex, Salton, etc.). There are several grain crackers on the market that are made to crack from coarse to fine, but will not produce fine flour.

If you like Cream of Wheat, or Cream of Rice cereals, you'll be amazed at how much better they taste when using freshly ground grains. Using my seed mill, I grind grains until all have been cracked at least in half. I sift out the smaller pieces to use for creamy hot cereals and save the larger pieces for cracked grain cereals and salads.

To store, follow above instructions for flours.

BEAN, PEA AND LENTIL FLOURS

WHY GRIND BEANS, PEAS AND LENTILS?
Grinding legumes to a flour allows you to make "instant" soups, sauces, dips, sandwich fillings and gravies. In fact, these flours can be added to almost everything you cook or bake.

- When added to boiling water, bean, pea and lentil flours thicken in only 1 minute, and in 3 minutes are ready to eat! Soups take only 3 minutes to cook. It takes only 5 minutes to make "refried beans." Compare that to soaking beans overnight, then cooking for 1 hour to soften. Many dry beans take 3 hours or more to cook.
- Combining these flours with grains forms a complete protein.
- Beans ground to a flour are easier to digest. Most bean flour users say that have no problems with flatulence.
- Sneaky! No one will guess that the creamy, white gravy you're pouring over potatoes, pasta, meatless patties or cooked vegetables contains BEANS! Who can tell that the cookies or muffins they love contain BEANS? What a great way to provide increased nutrition for finicky eaters.

WHAT BEANS, PEAS AND LENTILS ARE BEST?
- For 3-minute fat-free white sauces, gravies, cream soup bases, I use all kinds of white beans, as well as green and yellow peas, red and green lentils.
- For brown gravies, I use pinto and kidney beans.
- For 5-minute fat-free bean dips, I use pinto, black, kidney and garbanzo beans.
- For thickenings, I use white beans (all kinds) and red lentils.
- In baking, I use any and all beans, peas and lentils.

WHAT TO GRIND?

My favorite flours are: small white or navy beans, red lentils, pinto beans, black beans, and green peas. Limas are fantastic, but have to be cracked first (using blender or seed grinder) to fit into the milling chamber.

CRACKING BEANS, PEAS AND LENTILS

Coarsely cracked beans, peas, and lentils cook in only 15 minutes. Beans make a great breakfast cereal when mixed with cracked wheat, oats and brown rice. Add these to brown rice for a delicious, complete protein pilaf. Add to soups for a "soup-er" quick cooking option.

SPROUTS

"Sprouts grow practically anywhere; flourish in any climate, during any season of the year; need neither soil nor sunshine; are ready for harvest in 2-5 days; taste delicious raw or cooked; have no waste; and are so nutritious that they are one of the most complete foods known to man, rivaling meat in protein and citrus fruits in vitamin C at a fraction of the cost." (Northrup King Co., Consumer Products Division)

Growing a "garden" of sprouts requires much less effort than traditional outdoor or window gardens. Rinsing and draining several different kinds of sprouts takes only about 15 minutes a day and can provide a large variety of fresh vegetables not available in markets...and all for just pennies a day.

SPROUTING ADDS ENZYMES

Sprouting changes the composition of dried beans and legumes so they can be easily digested with little or no cooking. The "gas" or flatulence many people experience when eating beans is caused by the indigestible carbohydrates and sugars they contain. Sprouting adds enzymes to help break these down.

SPROUTS ARE VALUABLE SOURCES OF VITAMINS, MINERALS, AND PROTEINS

Sprouted grains and beans increase in vitamins A, B and C, E, and K. Riboflavin and folic acid increase up to 13 times the original amount present in dry seeds. Two of the most important amino acids necessary for the body to manufacture proteins are lysine and tryptophan, which are increased significantly during sprouting. Vitamin C increases up to 600% in some cases. (*Great Tasting Health Foods,* by Robert Rodale.)

Leafy, green sprouts such as alfalfa, radish, clover, sunflower and buckwheat lettuce and wheat grass, contain a rich supply of chlorophyll, a valuable source of vitamin A and protein. Research conducted by Dr. Charles R. Shaw, M.D., professor of biology at the University of Texas System Cancer Center in Houston, indicates the possibility that chlorophyll prevents formation of carcinoma (cancer) in mice. "The chlorophyll appears to exert its inhibitory effect (up to 99 percent effective) by interfering with enzymes which activate the carcinogens." This information applies to uncooked sprouts.

Nutrients and volume increase during sprouting, but calories do not, making sprouts a good low-calorie addition to any meal, or even as a meal by themselves. Many people use a variety of sauces and dressings added to a generous serving of various sprouts for a super delicious, nutritious, sprout meal or snack. Many children love to eat cool, crisp, clover and alfalfa sprouts by the handful.

It is best to serve a wide variety of sprouts to ensure a balanced diet since no one type of sprout contains all the essential nutrients to maintain good health.

HEATING DESTROYS NUTRIENTS
Many nutrients are destroyed by heat, but most people don't get too excited about eating all their food raw, and many sprouted beans don't taste good when eaten raw. The easiest way to ensure a sufficient supply of nutrients when sprouts must be cooked is to serve a generous helping of raw sprouts at the same meal in salads, sandwiches, dips, drinks or as snacks.

SPROUTED BEANS ARE MORE "FRIENDLY"
Cooking sprouted beans at high temperatures destroys all enzymes, but the conversion of starches to sugars that occurs during sprouting still allows cooked beans to be digested easily. (Adding meat, or any animal product, to sprouted beans will still

cause some gas to be produced.) White beans (Small White, Navy, Lima, Soy, etc.), peas and lentils are less likely to produce gas and can often be substituted for pinto or red beans.

ALL SEEDS CONTAIN ANTI-TRYPSIN INHIBITORS

All seeds contain an anti-digestant enzyme, which impairs the body's ability to digest proteins. The enzyme is a natural preservative that lasts until the proper environmental conditions bring them to life. According to Ann Wigmore, Hippocrates Diet and Health Program, the soaking and sprouting process leaches out this enzyme. Dr. Hal Johnson of the Benson Institute, Provo, Utah, maintains that only cooking destroys the enzyme and the body's ability to digest protein could be impaired if only uncooked sprouts were eaten for more than 1 year's time.

While it is unlikely any of us would have to live exclusively on sprouts for a whole year, it is a possibility that we may have to depend on them heavily until the next outdoor growing season. One family lived exclusively on sprouts for three years and experienced improved health, with no sickness whatever during that time period. (Sprout Handbook, by Stuart Wheelwright)

YIELD INCREASES WHEN GRAINS AND BEANS ARE SPROUTED

In addition to adding important enzymes, increasing nutrition, and saving time and effort in preparing whole foods, sprouting increases the yield for even greater savings on your food budget. A 15-ounce can of cooked kidney beans contains only about 4 ounces (1/4 pound) of dry beans which could be purchased for only about 15 cents. Sprouting 4 ounces of dry kidney beans yields about 1 1/2 pounds!

MOST POPULAR TYPES OF SEEDS

ADZUKI BEANS - Similar to the mung bean in flavor and nutrition, this small, red bean is a favorite in sprouted salad mixes, omelets, sandwiches, or just eaten plain.

ALFALFA - In Arabic, alfalfa means "father of all food." This tender, surprisingly sweet sprout is rich in vitamins A, B, C, D, E, F, and K, and in minerals such as phosphorus, iron, calcium, potassium, magnesium, sodium, silicon, and many more. Alfalfa also contains at least 8 of the essential enzymes.

BARLEY - Sprouting barley adds a chewy texture to a green or sprout salad mixture. Source of iron, phosphorus, and potassium.

BUCKWHEAT- Popular as a pancake flour, the whole seed is easy to sprout and can be grown until the first leaves appear, then used as a delicious, mild salad green. Combined with alfalfa, it makes a pleasing salad base. High in vitamins A, B, C, and D.

CLOVER - A tastier cousin to alfalfa, with larger leaves. A source of calcium chromium, magnesium, phosphorous, and potassium.

GARBANZO BEANS - Excellent source of protein. This is my all-time favorite bean because it tastes so good raw and adds such great nutrition to soups, sandwiches, dips, breads, and gravies.

MUNG BEANS - The crunchy, tasty mung bean is probably the most widely used of all sprouts. It is a favorite at salad bars and in many oriental recipes. Mung sprouts can be eaten after 2-3 days of sprouting, or can be sprouted under pressure for 5-7 days to produce long, juicy sprouts. They taste great either raw or cooked. Mung beans are also high in calcium, magnesium, phosphorus, and vitamins A, C, and E.

KIDNEY BEANS, PINTO BEANS and MISC. BEANS - Sprouting increases the already impressive amounts of vitamins, minerals, and protein. Sprouted kidney and pinto beans make wonderful "gas-free" chili, burritos, and bean dips.

LENTILS - With the flavor of freshly-ground mild black pepper, lentil sprouts are rich in iron and the B vitamins. They are delicious raw or cooked and because of their fresh, mild flavor, can be added to almost any recipe.

OATS - Sprouted oats are mild-tasting and an excellent addition to soups or salads. They can be used to make an excellent sprouted grain cereal or bread.

PEAS - Sprouted peas taste just like fresh peas from the garden! Add to soups and stews and cook only about 2 minutes for freshest flavor. Contains vitamin C, calcium and potassium.

QUINOA - This ancient grain is noted for its high protein. It sprouts 1/4" during the 4-hour soaking process and to 1" in only one day! It's literally "bursting" with goodness! This mild sprout is excellent in salads, sandwich fillings, or just plain!

RADISH- High in potassium and vitamin C, just one single sprout has the zesty flavor of an entire garden radish.

SOYBEANS - Ounce for ounce, the soybean contains twice as much protein as meat, four times that of eggs, twelve times that of milk. A complete protein even before sprouting, it is loaded with vitamins A, B, C, E, minerals and lecithin. One-half cup of the sprouts contains as much vitamin C as 6 glasses of orange juice! Soybeans can be sprouted under pressure, like mung beans, to produce long, succulent sprouts.

SUNFLOWER- Containing up to 50% protein, sunflower sprouts are also rich in vitamins B, D, and E as well as many minerals and "good" fats. A great source of instant energy. Sprouted sunflower seeds make an excellent breakfast drink when blended with fruit or fruit juices.

WHEAT- High in vitamins B, C, E, and minerals, the vitamin E content of wheat triples during the sprouting process, making it one of man's best sources for this important vitamin. When you sprout wheat for 3 days (including soaking time) you add to the wheat: enzymes, amino acids and additional vitamins and minerals.

DIRECTIONS FOR SPROUTING

Supplies needed:

❦ **Sprouting containers.** *Wide mouth quart jars* for alfalfa and other small, leafy greens, and easy to sprout seeds like adzuki, mung, peas, lentils, wheat, sunflower, barley, and oats; *trays* for green "lettuces" and grasses, and larger beans that sour easily.

❦ **Sprouting lids** (available at health food or preparedness stores), **fabric netting,** or a piece of **fiberglass screen** to cover jar opening. (In dry climates, a piece of nylon stocking works well.)

❦ **Sprouting seeds.** Organically grown seeds sprout the best for me. Any seed capable of growing into a plant will sprout.

The chart below will give you approximate amounts to use and how long the sprouting process should take. Times vary depending on age of seed and room temperature.

Type	Amount	Soaking Time	Sprouting Time	Yield
Alfalfa, quinoa, clover, radish, cress, or cabbage	2 T.	4 hrs.	5-7 days	2 c.
Grains, beans, peas, lentils, pumpkin, or sunflower	1/2 c.	10-12 hrs.	2-3 days	1 1/2 c.
Mung or soy (long)	1 c.	10-12 hrs.	5-6 days	4 c.
Wheat (for grass)	1 c.	10-12 hrs.	5-6 days	3 c.
Sunflower, or buck- wheat (for lettuce)	1 c.	10-12 hrs.	5-6 days	2 c.

Advance Preparation:

❦ **BUY FRESH SEEDS.** Fresh seeds tend to sprout faster and germinate better than those stored for long periods of time. Fresh seeds of all types are always easier to sprout, especially if they are from the current year's crop. Older seeds, especially beans, are usually slow to sprout and many in a batch will turn slimy and refuse to sprout. If you plan to buy large quantities of seeds for sprouting, ask for a sample and sprout a small amount first to test freshness. (If your stored beans or grains don't sprout, grind them to a flour and use for thickening or baking, or cook them whole.)

❦ **ROTATE YOUR SEED STORAGE.** Using sprouts often and buying a fresh supply of sprouting seeds each year will ensure best results.

❦ **For long-term storage, "AERATE" STORED SEEDS EVERY YEAR.** Dry seeds are "alive," but dormant. They "breathe" at a very slow rate, giving off carbon dioxide, so they need fresh oxygen periodically. If you choose to store sprouting seeds only for use in emergencies, Connie Nielsen of Life Sprouts, recommends pouring seeds out of, and then back into, their storage containers once every year or two.

❦ **START FRESH SPROUTS OFTEN.** One of the best reasons to sprout is be able to enjoy foods that are fresh and **full** of essential nutrients. Most seeds reach maturity after 2-5 days of sprouting. The vitamin C and enzyme levels begin to decrease after that time, so start small batches of sprouts often, rather than growing a huge batch and storing it in the refrigerator. I like to start a small amount of a different seed each day, in addition to my favorites that I sprout about twice a week. If I end up with too many sprouts to use raw, I freeze all but the green, leafy ones to use later in cooking.

Ready, Set, GO!
1. Sort and soak dry seeds. All seeds should be sorted, removing broken seeds and small pieces of debris. Place in a quart jar. Place sprouting lid or fabric (see suggestions above) over the top of the jar. If using fabric, secure with a jar ring or wide elastic band. Rinse seeds well, then pour off water and add soaking water— twice as much water as you have seeds. (Because of the excess salt

in softened water, and the chlorine in city water, it is best to use purified water for soaking and rinsing.)

2. After soaking, pour off water and drain well. Whether you leave seeds in the jar or transfer to a tray, tipping the container slightly will help seeds drain better. Most failures at sprouting occur because seeds are not drained properly. (After soaking most **beans,** pour onto sprouting tray and remove any seeds that have not expanded and are still hard; they will **not** sprout.) When no water drips from sprouts, roll jar so that most seeds coat sides of jar. To sprout in trays, spread seeds evenly, drain well, and cover with a lid or cloth to retain moisture and keep out light. Move to a warm (about 70°F) place and rinse with lukewarm water 2 times a day (or just often enough to keep moist for small seeds like alfalfa) until sprouts have reached the desired length.

3. Harvesting. Any seed CAN be eaten when the sprout has pushed through the outer shell of the seed. Most grains and beans and larger seeds are best when the sprout is as long as the seed. For instructions on growing "lettuce," wheat grass, and long, fat bean sprouts, see *Natural Meals in Minutes*, pp. 84-85.

4. "Greening." When leaves have appeared on small seeds like alfalfa, and sprouts are about 1" long, place jar in a light place (not in direct sunlight) to "green" for 3-4 hours, allowing the chlorophyll to develop.

5. "De-hulling." After "greening," put sprouts into a gallon jar or large pitcher and fill with water. The hulls will sink to the bottom or float to the top. Skim off floating hulls, then pour off water while lifting sprouts to top of the jar to allow water and hulls at the bottom of the container to pour off freely.

6. Storing Sprouts. Like any fresh vegetable, nutrients in sprouts deteriorate as soon as the sprout has reached maturity, usually within 2-3 days. Rather than grow large quantities of sprouts to store in the refrigerator for a week or more, start small quantities of fresh sprouts every few days. Check sprouts carefully, and if any mold appears on any type of sprouts, do not eat.

Store sprouted seeds in a covered container with paper toweling on the bottom and between layers. Use within 4-5 days. Sprouted beans and grains can be frozen for later use. Mung and soy beans that are sprouted to about 2" long turn limp when thawed, but can still be used in cooking. I put 2-cup portions of sprouted grains or legumes in quart zip-loc bags, force out excess air, then stack flattened bags in the freezer where they store well for 1-2 months.

HOW TO GROW SPROUTS IN COLD WEATHER

How would you grow sprouts if you didn't have any electricity in the wintertime? What if your house is cooler than the recommended sprouting temperature of 70°F?

Sprouts will still **grow** in cold weather, even in the refrigerator, but growth will be slower. In case of a power outage, you can "incubate" them by setting them in their jars or trays inside a "cooler," with 1-2 covered jars of boiling water set in the center. Place lid on top. The water may need to be reheated one or more times each day. A heavy cardboard box or plastic bucket or tub, wrapped in a mylar blanket or covered with heavy foil, will also work well to provide a warmer sprouting environment.

POPULAR USES FOR SPROUTS

Since many vitamins, minerals, and enzymes are destroyed in cooking, try to use the tender raw sprouts in uncooked recipes whenever possible, or add to cooked foods just before serving. Use them in drinks and smoothies, omelets, meat loaves, patties, in bread dough, casseroles, stir-fry, salads, or as "lettuce" in sandwiches.

■■■■■ FOOD COMBINING CHART ■■■■■

For best digestion, do NOT combine PROTEINS with STARCHES. Eat cooked FRUITS alone.

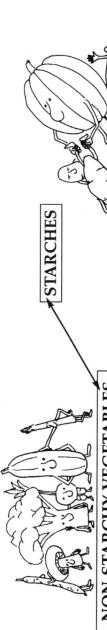

NON-STARCHY VEGETABLES

(all leafy veggies and sprouted seeds, grains, legumes, nuts; asparagus, beets, broccoli, cauliflower, cabbage family, celery, green beans, mushrooms, zucchini, and all summer squashes)

STARCHES

Starchy Vegetables

(carrots, potatoes, winter squash, yams)

Grains

(All breads, pasta, cooked cereals, cakes, cookies - amaranth, barley, buckwheat, corn, millet, oats, quinoa, rice, rye, spelt, triticale, wheat)

Legumes

(All beans - adzuki, black, blackeyed, garbanzo, great northern, kidney, lima, mung, peanuts, pinto, red, soy. All peas and lentils)

PROTEINS

Proteins

(gluten, soy products, tofu, tempeh, TVP, meats, fish and dairy products)

Nuts & Seeds

(almonds, cashews, filberts, flax, pecans, pine nuts, pumpkin, sesame, sunflower, walnuts)

FRUITS

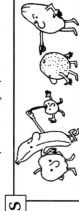

(apples, apricots, avocados, bananas, berries, dates, grapes, kiwi, lemon, mango, melons, nectarine, orange, papaya, peach, pear, pineapple)

©1998, Natural Meals In Minutes • www.naturalmeals.com

FOOD COMBINING GUIDELINES

- Raw fruits digest in 20 minutes; raw vegetables in 2 hours; proteins in 4 hours. A cooked meal combining all of these takes 12-24 hours! This extended transit time causes foods to ferment, creating indigestion and an extra burden on the body's eliminative organs.

- Eat raw, **Non-Starchy Vegetables** at the beginning of each cooked meal to add essential enzymes for digestion and to give your body the "raw materials" it needs to be able to heal.

- Make sure to have at least one raw meal each day to replenish your "enzyme bank account."

- Do NOT combine **Proteins** and **Starches.***

- Eat cooked **Fruits alone.** (Raw fruits combine well with ANY other raw food.)

*Note: SMALL quantities of protein foods (a garnish, rather than the main course) can be added to vegetable meals, such as chicken or tofu added to stir-fried vegetables, veggieburgers, rice and bean burritos, etc.

WELL-COMBINED COOKED MEALS

STARCHES + NON-STARCHY VEGETABLES
Rice and Bean-Filled Tacos with lettuce and tomatoes

◆

Bean and Rice Veggie Soup, Bread Sticks, and Green Salad

◆

Grain & Garden Burger made with rice, beans, onions, green peppers, and served with a raw Green Salad

◆

Pizza (made with tomato sauce, red and green peppers, olives, onions, garlic, mushrooms) and Green Salad

◆

Baked Potato with White Bean Gravy, Carrots, Green Salad

PROTEINS + NON-STARCHY VEGETABLES
Tossed Salad topped with alfalfa, lentil and mung bean sprouts, almonds and chicken or gluten strips

◆

Breaded Baked Tofu or Chicken Strips, broccoli and cauliflower

COMBINING RAW FOODS

- **ANY raw food combines well with ANY other raw food from ANY category.**

- **To activate enzymes**, whole raw grains, seeds, and legumes should be sprouted; nuts should be soaked at least 3 hours. Add to raw fruit breakfasts or raw veggie lunches to supply protein, "good" fat and starch.

- **Fruit Smoothies and whole meal salads** are quick and easy to prepare, very satisfying, and supply your body with readily available energy and nutrients.

Vegetable Salad Ideas - Fresh greens with grapes, carrots, sprouts (clover, sunflower seeds, wheat and lentils)

Fruit Salad Ideas - Serve on fresh lettuce or leafy sprouts - apples, grapes, banana, mango, pineapple, soaked almonds, and topped with sprouted wheat, barley, oats, or quinoa.

©1998, Natural Meals In Minutes • www.naturalmeals.com

Natural Food Pyramid

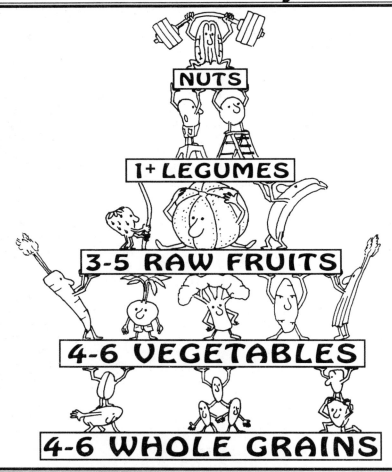

NUTS

1+ LEGUMES

3-5 RAW FRUITS

4-6 VEGETABLES

4-6 WHOLE GRAINS

SERVING SIZES: 2 oz. of nuts or nut butters (optional), 1/2 c. of all fruits, legumes, grains (1 slice bread), and vegetables (1 c. of raw, leafy veggies).

- Start each cooked meal with raw veggies and eat most fruits and veggies raw to supply vitamins, minerals and enzymes for digestion and healing.
- Combine grains and legumes for complete plant proteins.
- Eat most grains whole or cracked, not as bread or pasta.
- Include 1 c. dark green veggies each day to supply iron.
- Use meats and protein foods sparingly, as garnishes.
- Make sure to have at least one raw meal a day.
- Do not combine proteins and starches.
- DO sprout legumes to eliminate gas.

RAW!

RAW!

RAW!

NATURAL FOOD PYRAMID

NUTS AND SEEDS (Optional)
Eat 1-2 servings a day if you do NOT eat animal products.

Raw or sprouted nuts and many seeds are an important addition to the basic four foods, especially it you are not eating animal products. They supply essential protein, fiber and fat — the GOOD kind — as well as essential enzymes. **Serving size:** 2 ounces of nuts, high-fat seeds, or nut butters.

LEGUMES
Eat 1 or more servings a day.

Legumes (beans, peas, and lentils) are good sources of soluble fiber, protein, iron, calcium, zinc, and B vitamins. This group also includes all sprouted beans, baked and refried beans, gluten, soy milk, tempeh, tofu, and texturized vegetable protein (TVP). **Serving size:** 1/2 cup cooked (or sprouted) beans, gluten, tofu or tempeh; 8 ounces soy milk   If you choose to have fish and poultry, serving size is 2-3 ounces.   (If you are not including fish and poultry in your diet, be sure to include a supplement or a good source of vitamin B12, such as brewer's yeast.)

RAW FRUITS
Eat 3-5 servings a day of raw fruits to supply healing and digestive enzymes.

Fruits are rich in vitamins, fiber, vitamin C, and beta-carotene. Be sure to include at least one serving each day of fruits that are high in vitamin C (citrus fruits, melons, and strawberries). Choose whole fruit over fruit juices, which do not contain very much fiber. **Serving size:** 1 medium piece of fruit, about 1/2 cup; 6 oz. juice.

VEGETABLES
Eat 4-6 servings a day (most raw) and at LEAST 1 serving of green, leafy vegetables.

Vegetables are packed with vitamins and minerals. They provide vitamin C, beta-carotene, riboflavin, iron, calcium, fiber, and other nutrients. Dark green, leafy vegetables such as broccoli, collards, kale, mustard and turnip greens, spinach, chicory, or bok choy are especially good sources of these important nutrients, as well as a good source of protein. Dark yellow and orange vegetables such as carrots, winter squash, sweet potatoes, and pumpkin supply the antioxidant, beta-carotene. Include generous portions of raw and *colorful* vegetables in your diet for disease-fighting enzymes and antioxidants. **Serving size:** 1 cup raw leafy vegetables (lettuce, cabbage, spinach); 1/2 cup other raw or cooked vegetables (carrots, celery, potatoes, broccoli).

WHOLE GRAINS
Eat 4-6 servings a day (1-2 as breads, pasta)

This group includes all grains (amaranth, brown rice, bulgur, buckwheat, corn, millet, oats, quinoa, rye, spelt, triticale, wheat), all breads, pasta, hot or cold cereals. Eat mostly whole grains rather than grains ground to a flour, such as breads, pasta, etc. Sprout grains for increased enzymes, vitamins, and minerals. Build your evening meal around hearty grains (& legumes); grains are rich in fiber and complex carbohydrates, as well as protein, B vitamins, and zinc. **Serving size:** 1/2 cup hot cereal; 1 ounce dry cereal; 1 slice whole grain bread.   This category should be combined with vegetables to maintain stable blood sugar (whole grains with chopped vegetables; sandwiches made with LOTS of lettuce and sliced cucumbers; pasta with vegetables; barley vegetable soup).

Try eating primarily from these Essential Food Groups,
with as many raw foods as possible. You'll discover a healthier way to live!

Natural Foods Shopping List

Supplements
- ❏ acidophilus powder
- ❏ aloe vera juice
- ❏ brewer's yeast
- ❏ C-Crystals (vitamin C powder)
- ❏ flaxseed oil-Barlean's
- ❏ liquid chlorophyll
- ❏ spirulina or barley green

Flavorings - Sweeteners
- ❏ carob powder
- ❏ coconut extract
- ❏ honey
- ❏ malted milk powder
- ❏ maple extract
- ❏ orange extract
- ❏ pecan nut flavoring
- ❏ pure maple syrup
- ❏ rum flavoring - artificial
- ❏ vanilla extract

Fruits - fresh / frozen
- ❏ apples
- ❏ applesauce, unsweetened
- ❏ apricots
- ❏ avocado
- ❏ bananas
- ❏ blackberries
- ❏ blueberries
- ❏ cantaloupe
- ❏ casaba melon
- ❏ honeydew melon
- ❏ kiwi fruit
- ❏ lemon
- ❏ lime
- ❏ mango
- ❏ pineapple
- ❏ pineapple chunks, in juice
- ❏ pineapple, crushed, in juice
- ❏ oranges
- ❏ papayas
- ❏ peaches
- ❏ pears
- ❏ plums
- ❏ red grapes
- ❏ raisins
- ❏ raspberries
- ❏ red apples
- ❏ strawberries
- ❏ watermelon

100% Fruit Juices
- ❏ Black Cherry-Knudsen
- ❏ Apricot Nectar-Knudsen
- ❏ cranberry
- ❏ fruit punch
- ❏ fresh-squeezed grapefruit
- ❏ lemon
- ❏ Vita Juice-Simply Nutritious
- ❏ Pineapple Juice-Del Monte
- ❏ papaya nectar

100% Fruit Juice Concentrates
- ❏ orange
- ❏ apple
- ❏ grape
- ❏ creamed papaya

Dole 100% Fruit Juice Concentrates
- ❏ Country Raspberry
- ❏ Mountain Cherry
- ❏ Pineapple Orange
- ❏ Pineapple-Orange Banana
- ❏ Pineapple-Orange Strawberry
- ❏ Pineapple

Welch's 100% Fruit Juice Concentrates (these 100% juices DO NOT contain sulfites)
- ❏ White Grape
- ❏ White Grape Cranberry
- ❏ White Grape Peach
- ❏ White Grape Raspberry

100% Fruit Spreads
- ❏ blueberry
- ❏ apricot
- ❏ strawberry

Whole Grains or Grain Flours
- ❏ amaranth
- ❏ barley
- ❏ buckwheat
- ❏ corn
- ❏ millet
- ❏ oats
- ❏ quinoa
- ❏ brown rice
- ❏ rye
- ❏ spelt
- ❏ triticale
- ❏ wheat

Natural Foods Shopping List, Cont'd

Legumes
- [ ] anasazi beans
- [ ] adzuki beans
- [ ] black beans
- [ ] black lentils
- [ ] blackeyed peas
- [ ] fava beans
- [ ] garbanzo beans
- [ ] great northern beans
- [ ] green lentils
- [ ] green peas
- [ ] kidney beans
- [ ] lima beans
- [ ] mung beans
- [ ] navy beans
- [ ] pea beans
- [ ] peanuts/peanut butter
- [ ] pink beans
- [ ] pinto beans
- [ ] red beans
- [ ] red lentils
- [ ] small white beans
- [ ] soy beans
- [ ] tofu & soy products
- [ ] yellow peas

Milk - Dry
- [ ] non-fat powdered milk- non-instant

Milks - Non-Dairy (liquid or powder)
- [ ] almond milk-Pacific Foods
- [ ] oat milk
- [ ] Better Than Milk, rice or soy
  - [ ] vanilla [ ] plain
- [ ] soy beverage, non fat-WestSoy
- [ ] Rice Dream-Imagine Foods
- [ ] rice milk, fat free, plain
- [ ] soy milk, regular, lite or fat-free
- [ ] Rice Moo-Sovex
- [ ] Soy Moo-Health Valley

Nuts & Seeds
- [ ] alfalfa seeds
- [ ] almonds
- [ ] broccoli seeds
- [ ] cabbage seeds
- [ ] cashews
- [ ] clover seeds
- [ ] filberts

- [ ] flax seeds
- [ ] pecans
- [ ] pine nuts
- [ ] poppy seeds
- [ ] pumpkin seeds
- [ ] radish seeds
- [ ] brown sesame seeds
- [ ] sunflower seeds
- [ ] walnuts

Nut/Seed Butters
- [ ] almond butter
- [ ] cashew butter
- [ ] tahini (sesame seed butter)

Protein Powders
- [ ] Nature's Life Pro-Life Soy
- [ ] Nutribiotic Organic Rice
- [ ] Naturade Vegetable

Bouillons
- [ ] Better Than Bouillon Superior
      Touch Vegetarian Vegetable,
      Beef or Chicken
- [ ] HerbOx bouillons - without MSG

Tofu
- [ ] any brand - choose from
      low-fat or regular
- [ ] lite tofu, firm-Mori-nu (my favorite)

Vegetables
- [ ] asparagus
- [ ] beans, green
- [ ] beets and greens
- [ ] cabbage family
- [ ] carrots
- [ ] ginger root
- [ ] mint leaves
- [ ] mushrooms
- [ ] parsley
- [ ] potatoes
- [ ] red and green bell peppers
- [ ] spinach
- [ ] squash, all types
- [ ] sweet potatoes
- [ ] Swiss chard

PUBLICATIONS WORTH ORDERING

NATURAL MEALS PUBLISHING

For a distributor nearest you, call **1-888-232-6706**

www.naturalmeals.com   E-mail: info@naturalmeals.com

COUNTRY BEANS *by Rita Bingham*

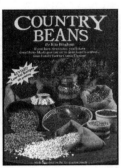

Nearly 400 quick, easy meatless bean recipes with over 110 bean flour recipes, including FAST, fat-free 3-minute bean soups and 5-minute bean dips. Learn how to grind your own bean, pea and lentil flours, or where to purchase them. Most recipes are wheat-free, gluten-free, and dairy-free. Recipes for every meal of the day. Guaranteed to change the way you use beans! **$14.95**

NATURAL MEALS IN MINUTES *by Rita Bingham*

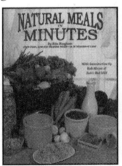

Over 300 quick, high-fiber, low-fat, meatless recipes using wholesome storage foods. All meals made in 30 minutes or less!
- FAST meals using Grains and Beans
- Bean, Seed and Grain Sprouts
- 3-minute fat-free Powdered Milk Cheeses

Each recipe lists nutritional information. (Learn sneaky tricks for adding extra fiber to every meal.) Guaranteed to please! **$14.95**

THE NEW PASSPORT TO SURVIVAL *by Bingham/Dickey*

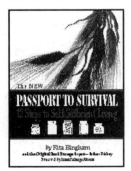

12 Steps To Self-Sufficient Living. How to survive natural, man-made, or personal disasters. Twelve easy steps to becoming self-sufficient, without panic! Includes quick mixes and heart-smart recipes to put you on the road to better health.

Learn what to store and why, where to store, and how to use what you store on a daily basis. **Learn what nutritious foods to store for only $150 per year per person!** **$15.95**

Quick WHOLESOME FOODS video with recipe booklet
by Bingham and Moulton

Whether you're preparing for emergencies, or just want to make quick, inexpensive meals, you'll learn to make easy recipes:

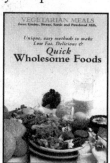

- Light, fluffy, 100% whole wheat breads
- Meatless spicy sausage, and thick steaklets
- Breakfasts, snacks and desserts using Whole Grains and Seeds
- Non-fat 3-minute powdered milk cheeses, including Country Chicken Fried Steak - mouthwatering and irresistable!
- 3-minute no-fat bean soups and cream sauces

Make delicious, nutritious, vegetarian meals in 30 minutes or less. 65 minutes, VHS **$29.95**

1-2-3 SMOOTHIES *by Rita Bingham*

123 Quick Frosty Drinks - Delicious AND Nutritious!

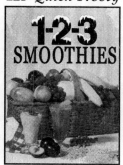

Is there one perfect breakfast—afternoon snack—meal-on-the-run—or one perfect way to sneak nutritious vitamins and other important nutrients into a finicky eater? YES! It's a 1-2-3 Smoothie! These energy-boosting, nutritious drinks are the hottest COOL healthy treats ever! 100% natural ingredients - no sugar, preservatives, artificial sweeteners, or added fat. **$14.95**

SAUCES, SEASONINGS AND NATURAL FOODS *Bingham*

Over 200 recipes using whole foods to create healthy sauces, seasonings and delicious, nutritious meals—from home-style to gourmet! Meals ready in a FLASH! Most recipes are gluten-free, dairy-free, and have no added fats or refined sugars.

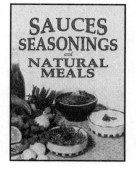

*Salads and Dressings • Spice Blends
Seasoning Mixes • Quick Mixes • Fruit Sauces,
Pasta Sauces • Marinades • Dips • Spreads
Fat-Free Gravies and MUCH more!*

Nutritional data included for each quick, easy recipe. **$15.95** *Available February, 2000*

OTHER VALUABLE PUBLICATIONS

Cookin' With Home Storage, by Tate and Layton. Over 700 recipes - Down home cookin' with the basics, Dutch oven cooking, sprouting, natural beauty & personal care. **$14.95** + $3.50 s&H. Call (435) 835-8283. *(Note: Some recipes contain processed oils and refined sugar.)*

Dynamic Health, and **An Apple A Day,** by Dr. M. Ted Morter. Call 1-800-281-4450 for more information on how to monitor your level of health by testing your body's reaction to acid foods.

Enzymes and Enzyme Therapy, by Dr. Anthony Cichoke. Keats Publishing, New Canaan, Connecticut.

Food Enzymes: The Missing Link to Radiant Health, by Humbart Santillo. Hohm Press, Prescott, AZ.

Feed Your Kids Right, and **Foods For Healthy Kids,** by Dr. Lendon Smith. Dell Publishing, New York, 10017. Illness, hyperactivity, and even stress can be prevented if your child eats right.

Food & Behavior, by Barbara Reed Stitt. Natural Press, P. O. Box 730, Manitowoc, WI 54221-0730. Learn the biochemical connection between the foods we eat, behavior and health.

The Amazing Wheat Book, by LeArta Moulton. This unique cook book can save you time and money. Find delicious, wholesome, fast recipes. Whole wheat breads, rolls, muffins, crackers, chips, soups, salads, and more. Learn how to make wheat meat for 1/4th the cost of meat (meatballs, jerky, veggie burger, sausage & even pet food.) Prepare your own seasoning & sauce blends. Saves you money & eliminates preservatives. *(Note: Some recipes in this book contain refined sugar.)* **$14.95** + $3.50 s&H. Call (888) 554-3727.

The Food Storage Bible, by Jayne Benkendorf. A quick, easy reference guide for selecting thousands of healthful grocery products free of harmful preservatives. **$16.95** Call (800) 580-1414.

15 Minute Storage Meals, A Cookbook For the Busy Person, by Jayne Benkendorf. Learn the "Fabulous 30" high energy foods for better health, plus 30 tasty, low fat recipes for meals in only 15 minutes. Incluces a one-month storage shopping list using items listed in The Food Storage Bible. **$12.95** Call (800) 580-1414.